HEALING IN THE DANCE

Healing
in the Dance

An investigation into the therapeutic
nature of dance

MARTIN BLOGG

KINGSWAY PUBLICATIONS
EASTBOURNE

Biblical quotations are from
the Holy Bible: New International Version,
© International Bible Society 1973, 1978, 1984.

Front cover photo by Martin Blogg

British Library Cataloguing in Publication Data

Blogg, Martin H.
   Healing in the dance.
   1. Medicine. Dance therapy
   I. Title
   616.89'1655

ISBN 0-86065-478-8

Printed in Great Britain for
KINGSWAY PUBLICATIONS LTD
Lottbridge Drove, Eastbourne, E Sussex BN23 6NT by
Richard Clay Ltd, Bungay, Suffolk.
Typeset by Nuprint Ltd, Harpenden, Herts AL5 4SE

To

Alison Charles

Christian Dance Ministries

and

Springs Dance Company

—all of whom I have had the
privilege of serving with in Christian dance

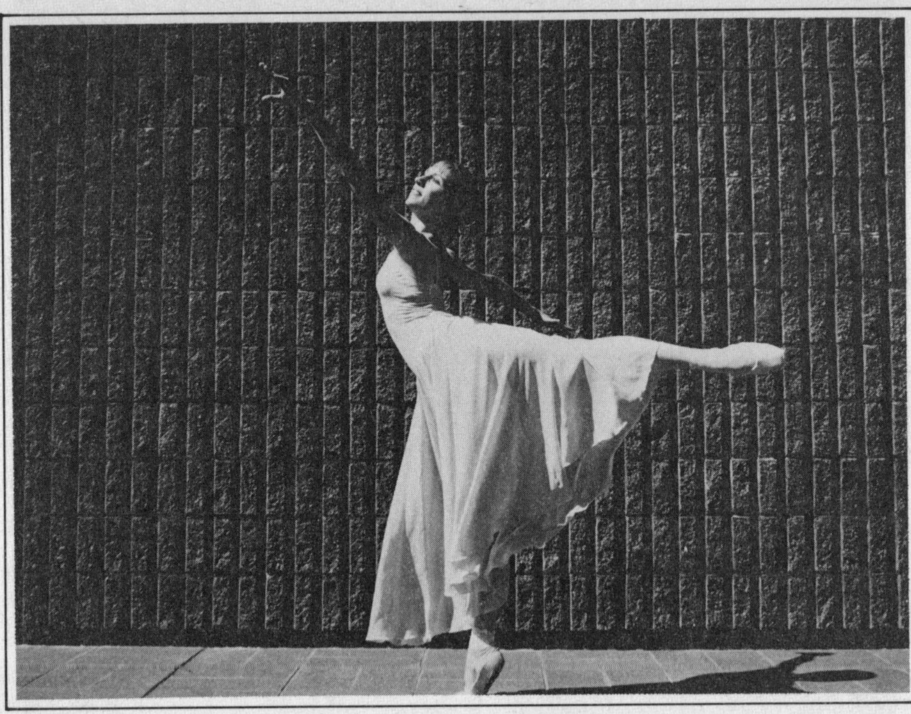

'Whoever lives by the truth, comes into the light' (Jn 3:21).

Contents

Introduction

> I was a student of theology who became a dancer — I did not
> abandon religion for dancing, but sought it in the dance.
>
> *Ted Shawn — dancer*

Most justifications for dance within the contemporary
Christian faith have been made largely from the point of view
of worship and communication. The notion of dance as a
means to health and healing, although one of its oldest and
original justifications, has received much less attention. As is
evidenced by the number of books coming out on this subject,
the topic of 'healing' itself is receiving some considerable
attention within the church at this time. Indeed, healing is
experiencing something of a revival as more and more churches
seek to establish a healing ministry, thus beginning to restore
to its rightful place one of the three fundamental aspects of
Christ's ministry of reconciliation on this earth: teaching,
preaching and healing (Mt 4:23). It is within this renewed
and growing interest by the church in health and healing and
also within advances made in contemporary medicine that I
wish to contribute, showing in both theoretical and practical
terms that dance, and the allied arts of music and drama,
constitute an immensely rich source of health and healing.

The primary focus of this book is not on dance for its own
sake, but rather on health and healing — mental, physical,

emotional and social well being. I see dance as a means to that end as it relates to the ministry of healing within the church. So this is not a treatise on aesthetics but a discussion about the nature and conditions of dance as a means to health and healing.

This book is also not concerned primarily with health and healing, sickness and dis-ease, in the institutionalised or hospitalised sense of the term, although undoubtedly there is much here of relevance to such states of dis-ease and, indeed, much of the enclosed research comes from such sources. Rather, my concern is with the more normal, everyday, dis-eased people, who make up the vast majority of our society, and of the church particularly as they take up the cross and pursue the Christian faith.

The book does not set out to represent an all-embracing, thoroughly detailed and scholarly study of dance as therapy and a means to health and healing, though it is, I hasten to add, based upon a disciplined concern for research gathered from medical and social science. Rather, it is written for the non-specialist in health and healing, and written, I hope, in a way that is readable, meaningful and relevant. It is written in order to explain in both theoretical and practical terms something of the contemporary thinking about the nature and conditions of dance as 'recreation' and 'therapy'. Although it is aimed at the Christian dancer and those interested in dance, it is by no means concerned exclusively with the dancer or dance. Health and healing are the concern of everybody, so much here is relevant to every member of the congregation—young and old, dancer and non-dancer.

In writing this book my two main concerns were:
(1) The nature and conditions of dance as a means to health and healing as seen within (a) Scripture; (b) 'medicine'—in the broadest sense of the term, including both the medical and social sciences; and (c) the broader ministry of the church.
(2) The crucial and fundamental importance of health—

mental, physical, emotional and social—as it relates to the individual dancer within Christian dance, and as it relates to the dance group as a Christian healing ministry.

I have drawn on three sources:

1. Personal experience

It is, first of all, based on the practical everyday experience of working within professional Christian dance, being 'on the road' and 'in the market place', intimately involved on a day-to-day basis, working out my faith and ministry in personal and professional terms. What I have written arises *not* out of merely listening to the word—which can result in self-deception—but out of doing it (Jas 1:22). It is a knowledge which comes from the heart (Mk 7:6). As Tozer once said, 'Truth that is not experienced is little less than error, and maybe equally as dangerous.' The truths shared in this writing are thoroughly rooted in Scripture and carefully substantiated where appropriate by medical and social research. But fundamentally they have been worked out and realised in first-hand everyday living.

The writing will, I hope, have an encouraging familiarity about it. It is in no sense a rarified theoretical abstraction, nor is it an idealistic super-spiritual fantasy. Quite the contrary. It is the expression of an ordinary, normal and 'healthy' dis-eased member of the faith who, over a long, hard-earned, sustained period of commitment within the ministry of Christian dance has begun to recognise and understand, in both theoretical and practical terms, something of the essential nature and paradox of Christian life as it relates to dance and health and healing. The Teacher who wrote Ecclesiastes says, 'There is a time to weep and a time to laugh, a time to mourn and a time to dance' (3:4). Joy and pain together go to make up life, and are two sides of the same coin. Our faith, while on the one hand promising great peace, joy and fulness of life, also brings with it, almost as a prerequisite, profound dis-ease and suffering, both personal and collective. This is, of course, what the message of the faith is all about. 'The way of the cross' is in no sense an easy or comfortable way—but it is *the* way, the only way as all Christians must, sooner or later, painfully come to know. Dis-ease is an inevitable part of human growth and development. It is as if in some mysterious way we have to experience pain and suffering in order to be healthy and whole.[1] Accordingly, this book on health and healing is very much to do with dis-ease, meaning dis-ease not simply of the body, but of the whole human be-ing,— mental, physical, emotional, social and spiritual. For the Christian, although there is no doubt that God wants us healthy and whole, free from sickness and dis-ease, and that this was the specific purpose of his coming to this earth (Jn 10:10), growth into this whole life can be painful. Scriptural truths are designed to set us free, but the process of becoming free involves some painful purging because of our sinful nature. Coming to understand this paradox of the faith, acknowledging our sickness and dis-ease and the truth of such statements as, 'The whole creation has been groaning' (Rom 8:22), 'There is no-one righteous, not even one' (Rom 3:10), 'For what I want to do I do not do' (Rom 7:15), is an important step to becoming healthy and whole. Once we are able to grasp these fundamental truths there is, I believe, an extraordinary liberation of mind, body, heart and spirit. This growing recognition, while it may not result in a more easy or comfortable journey, will reassure us that pain is a potentially healthy and positive part of our growth.

Anyone writing about health and healing, or concerned to bring about health and healing—religious or otherwise— must of necessity, for his sake and for the sake of those whom he seeks to serve, acknowledge first his own brokenness, dis-ease and inadequacy. This, I do now, wholeheartedly and with humility. As Thomas Merton wrote, 'Before a man can become a saint, he must first of all be a man in all the humanity and fragility of men's actual condition.[2] Before one can legitimately embark upon a healthy healing ministry, one must first have acknowledged and experienced something of this brokenness within 'the humanity and fragility' of human being. This is an essential prerequisite for such a ministry. Significantly the most effective healers are usually the wounded ones. 'The path of health and wholeness requires us to understand the paradoxes and conflicts of human being, accepting the task of writing the form of heaven with the energy of hell'.[3] From this growing recognition of our sinful nature and the pain and suffering that results from our struggles with our nature, there gradually emerges one of the most profound and primary qualifications for a ministry in healing—compassion. All too often in my experience the truth for many Christians is a truth that is written on tablets of stone and not experienced by the human heart (Mk 7:6). Compassion is at the heart of the Christian faith. It was at the heart of Jesus' ministry—witness his concern both for truth *and* love in his healing work. Compassion, as expressed in the Passion, is at the heart of truth and love. Compassion does not reside in propositional knowledge and legalistic truth. (Nor does it lie simply in good deeds in themselves.) Rather it resides *in*, and arises *from*, a wholehearted and practical experience of the word of God (Heb 4:12). It is not based on the written word by itself, but on the word and the personal experience of the heart, the experience of having fallen, of failure, of having been broken, and then of having been forgiven and redeemed—above all, of having been forgiven in the tender mercies of his compassion.

A full and proper knowledge and understanding of truth cannot be obtained simply by studying the written word alone. Knowledge *about* God has to be worked out and experienced in the 'full humanity and fragility of men's actual condition.' *How* we live our lives and realise these scriptural truths in our everyday living and loving will eventually lead us to the full and true nature of love and truth. Compassion, and the experiences from which it arises, is an essential and distinguishing element of all true love and is fundamental to a health and healing ministry, as we shall see most clearly when we come to discuss in detail the nature of dis-ease and suffering. The Christian is only perfect in God alone: that is in the sense of purity of intention and this is enjoined upon us by God (Mt 4:28). Any striving for perfection in terms of achievement is a mark of naivety and arrogance. Purity of intention is our hope as finite, fallible human beings. The man is perfect in faith who can come to God in the complete emptiness of his self-centred feelings and desires, without a glow of selfish aspiration, or with the weight of selfish thoughts, failures, negligence, straying or forgetfulness, and say to God, 'You are my refuge.' This must be the state of the Christian healer. But in spite of the 'mourning', that must of necessity be the Christian's lot, the faith is essentially a joy-full faith (Lk 4:18; Jn 10:10, 15:11). Throughout the Bible 'dancing' and 'mourning' go together, the former usually arising out of the latter, with joy always rising above all else.

Significantly, dancing is synonymous with giving thanks and praise, with being glad, rejoicing, feasting and merry-making. Dance in Scripture is never equated with suffering. It is clear from both Scripture and medicine that dancing has a very real contribution to make to health and healing. Accordingly, it has a very important place within this book and is represented in the practical dances of the third section of this book.

2. The needs of society and the church

My second source and motivation for writing arises out of the recognition of an ever-growing concern within society generally, and the church particularly, with regard to health and healing—especially the mental, emotional, social and spiritual aspects of human being which has frequently been neglected by traditional medicine with its inherited focus on pathology and physical disease rather than holistic health.

I have to admit that my own experiences within dance and the Christian faith, until recently at least, have been largely concerned with 'communication', with outreach and renewal, and the propagation of the faith. My major, if not exclusive emphasis, has been with professional dance skills, technique, vocabulary and choreography as they relate to worship and communication. Health and healing has not been an immediate concern, although I have for a long time recognised its potential importance. Only in the last two years or so have I come to recognise formally and deliberately such a ministry of dance and something of the extraordinary potential of expressive movement, together with its allied arts of music and drama. All this, I hasten to add, is not meant to undermine or underestimate in any way the power of dance as a means for communication in a much more general way. Rather, my concern for health and healing goes alongside such established developments within dance and the faith. Encouraged and supported by what I recognised as a need both within secular and religious 'medicine', and by what I have come to realise and acknowledge as an important concern within my own ministry, I was prompted to set out on an investigation into the community, educative and therapeutic aspects of dance as seen from within the disciplines of Scripture, medicine and dance. This book is the product of this journey.

3. Research findings

My third source comes, necessarily secondhand, from the research findings of medical and social science. Although I am a graduate in the social sciences with specialist interest in the social psychology of deviancy and illness, my primary professional qualifications and experience lie in dance, education, and the performing arts. You will understand, therefore, my professional obligation to refer to specialist sources of knowledge and understanding related to this area of study. The area of health and healing is a vast and complex inter-relation of many medical and social science disciplines including medicine, psychology/psychiatry, sociology, social psychology, physical education and sports medicine, recreation, health, anthropology, philosophy and history! I will be drawing upon the knowledge and research of such specialisms in my concern to develop a disciplined understanding of the nature and conditions of dance as a means to health and healing. In the majority of cases I have acknowledged the origins of my source, not simply in adherence to professional etiquette, but that the reader may be encouraged to probe more deeply into this relatively new subject. The study of dance as therapy, as any professional dance therapist will be the first to admit, is still very much in its infancy. There is still much to be done, much more to be discovered in both practical and theoretical terms.

This book sets out to encourage and support those concerned with dance as a means to health and healing. It sets out also, by implication, to question what I believe to be a predominantly elitist conception of dance — namely dance as 'high art' entertainment, the expression of a relatively few people performed by an even smaller minority. While I in no way wish to undermine or underestimate the recent encouraging growth of the dance audience, I do seriously want to question contemporary dance's narrow focus both in terms of forms and function. With respect to all that *is* happening in dance, I would seek to free dance from its present 'high art' exclusiveness, and begin to restore it to its original multidimensional and multifunctional position within community as a whole. I would like to see dance becoming once more a means of expression and communication for all people, for all occasions, and related to all aspects of life. But above all I would like to see it reappear as a means of community and health—mental, physical, emotional and social.

Martin Blogg
Wollaston College 1987

Notes

1. C S Lewis, *The Problem of Pain* (Fontana: London).
2. Thomas Merton, *Life in Holiness* (Image: London).
3. J A Sandford, *Healing and Wholeness* (Paulist Press, 1977).

PART 1

The Source of Health and Healing

I

The Fundamental Importance of Scripture

Any discussion of the nature and conditions of a ministry of health and healing must be rooted in Scripture. 'All Scripture is God-breathed and is useful for teaching, rebuking, correcting and training in righteousness' (2 Tim 3:16). We are nourished by God's word (Heb 5:12) which is 'sharper than any double-edged sword' (Heb 4:12). A ministry of health and healing must have a sound biblical base.

Basic to a Christian understanding of health and healing is a proper understanding of the nature of man and his relation to God.

The nature of man

The Bible clearly teaches that 'the earth is the Lord's, and everything in it' (Ps 24:1, see also Jn 1:3, Acts 17:24); and, as the Psalmist declared, we should 'know that the Lord is God. It is he who made us, and we are his' (Ps 100:3). From him comes our power to live each minute of the day and our work is valueless if not done in dependence on him.

Central to the Christian interpretation of the world and of man's place in it, is this biblical revelation of God's sovereignty and an all embracing purpose for his creation. All that 'is', depends on him, deriving its very existence from the ever creative God. [1]

20

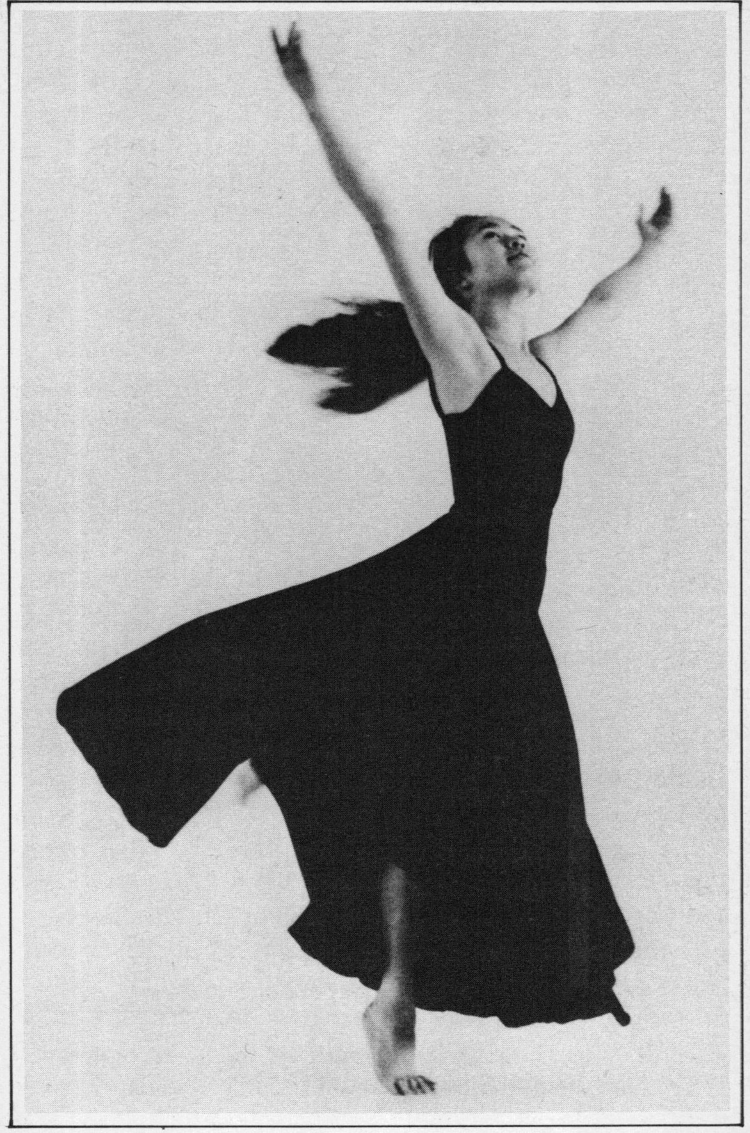

'Christ will be exalted in my body' (Phil 1:20).

Health and healing are related to the scriptural fact that we are creatures of God and in him we move and have our being. As creatures of the divine Creator, we are subject to his laws, and a proper knowledge and understanding of these laws is, therefore, essential to the knowledge of health and healing.

Jesus Christ reaffirmed these basic truths with regard to the nature of man and his relation to God. 'I bring you good news of great joy that will be for all the people,' proclaimed the angel (Lk 2:10). This great and glorious news is salvation and redemption, offered us through our Lord Jesus Christ. 'The Word became flesh, and made his dwelling among us' (Jn 1:14), and he came in order to rescue us 'from the dominion of darkness' and to bring us 'into the kingdom of the Son he loves' (Col 1:13). Jesus said that he had come in order that we might have life—and have it to the full (Jn 10:10). He gives us his peace (Jn 14:27) which in the Bible means not merely absence of worry, but health, wholeness and complete inner harmony. The life of health and healing represents a major thrust of the New Testament. It is intimately related to restoration, salvation and redemption. Jesus said, 'Whoever follows me will never walk in darkness, but [on the contrary] will have the light of life' (Jn 8:12). He was the bread of life and those who came to him would neither hunger nor thirst (Jn 6:35). By his power we were created, and by his love we were redeemed.

St Augustine wrote, 'My heart is restless, till it rest in thee.' The empty space, the dis-ease that is characteristic of so many hearts and minds today, is essentially a consequence and expression of this divorce between Creator and creature, between God and man. This dis-eased and empty space is uniquely shaped, and the only occupant that will fit it, fill it, and satisfy it is he who *is* love. (1 Jn 4:8). 'It may be said that man is instinctively religious, and he cannot be truly whole in soul, mind and body until he has come to this experience, until he has been touched by the reality of God'.[2]

Carl Jung also recognised the importance of God in healing the dis-eases of mankind. He wrote:

> During the past thirty years, people from all civilised countries of the earth have consulted me. I have treated many hundreds of patients . . . Among all my patients in the second half of life— that is to say, over thirty-five—there has not been one whose problem in the last resort was not that of finding a religious outlook on life. . . It seems to me that, side by side with the decline of religious life, the neuroses grow noticeably more frequent. . . . In the last analysis it is argued then, real health of body and mind depends upon one's religious life.

H G Wells once said, 'Until a man has found God, he begins at no beginning, and works to no end!' Without him we can do nothing! (Jn 15:5). Only the fool says in his heart, there is no God! (see Ps 14:1), and it is only the fool who thinks that he is big enough or smart enough to violate the unchangeable laws of the eternal God and get away with it. As creatures of God, dependent upon God, we must base our lives upon the stability and dependability of God as expressed in the laws. When we disobey these laws we must expect to experience dis-ease, and no power makes us suffer other than ourselves. When we learn to live by these laws we will become free from many dis-eases. This is an extraordinary and profound truth which is becoming increasingly accepted within contemporary medicine. Although not always described in biblical terms, much research would confirm that obedience to such basic laws of Scripture would save us from a wide variety of dis-eases, and death![3] Much dis-ease in our society, it will be shown, derives very much from ignoring and underestimating the importance of these basic, God-given, natural laws.

We are *dependent* beings, created by God; we are dependent upon God. We are also finite. We are not autonomous, with all those rights and imagined powers that we arrogate to ourselves, but finite, dependent creatures whose very existence depends upon God Himself.[4]

Health and healing as recorded in Scripture

First, when Scripture talks about health and healing, it refers to something much broader and more profound than physical disease alone. When Psalm 67 talks of God's *saving health* being known among all nations, when Psalm 43 describes God as 'the *health* of my countenance' and when the general confession in the 1662 Anglican *Book of Common Prayer* says, 'there is no *health* in us', something more is meant than the mere absence of physical dis-ease. In Scripture health is synonymous with 'wholeness', and involves a balanced integration of mind, emotions, body, community and spirit, within the experience of salvation and redemption.

Secondly, while it is true that there is much sickness and disease in the world, it should be understood that according to Scripture this is not the will of God.

> God does not *will* disease. He may permit it in His universe just as in the same way He permits sin, but we should understand that it was not a part of His purpose and design. Sickness and disease are intrusions in God's creation, and it is only when we see them in these terms that we can begin to have a proper attitude towards them.[5]

Basic to any Christian view of health and healing must be Jesus' keynote words, recorded in John 10:10: 'I have come that they may have life and have it to the full.' Basic to the biblical understanding of God's purpose for mankind is the principle that life is meant to be good and enjoyed, and enjoyed to the full! And Jesus came that we might have this life.

Thirdly, even a casual reading of the gospels will convince

the reader that bringing health and healing was a significant part of Jesus' ministry. In contrast to the greater part of the Old Testament, the New is filled with practical healing, and Jesus is the healer par excellence. His ministry, alone, abounds with examples of his compassion and concern for healing and for health. Something like a third of the narrative of the gospels is taken up with recording stories of healing. This is not surprising when one considers that Jesus' ministry was a threefold one involving teaching, preaching and healing (Mt 4:23). When we look at our Lord's ministry it is clear that healing in its broadest sense was, *and still is*, the very essence of the gospel, the 'good news'. In his first recorded sermon, given at the synagogue of Nazareth, when he announced the purpose of being here on earth, he expressed his concern for the sick, the poor and broken hearted, the ignorant, the disabled and the oppressed (Lk 4:18, 19 cf Is 61:1).

'I have discovered,' writes Selwyn Hughes, 'that whenever you meet Jesus Christ in the Gospels, He is either on His way to heal someone who is sick, on His way back from someone who is sick, or is actually about to heal someone who is sick.'[6] It is a scriptural fact that he healed all who were sick, 'to fulfil what was spoken through the prophet Isaiah: "He took up our infirmities and carried our diseases"' (Mt 8:17). His concern was not just for broken bodies but rather for dis-eased *persons*. His precepts in the Sermon on the Mount, and elsewhere, dealing with human motives and the deep workings of the mind show that he was acutely aware of the place emotions, conflict, resentment, fear, hatred and the like have in the basis of dis-ease. Jesus clearly regarded dis-ease as a holistic phenomenon involving mind, body, emotions and relationships, and while he was always concerned to heal the body, he invariably paid close attention to the mind, emotions and spirit as well.

In considering all the various related meanings to health

and healing in scripture, J P Baker concludes,

> Taking all the words used for healing, health and salvation together we begin to obtain a notion of wholeness as meaning 'completeness', all-round health and life and strength, obtaining freedom from evil and its effects at every level of our personal being and in all our relationships.[7]

That is the goal to which God's saving purpose seeks to move us on. Wholeness is not just to make us well, it is to make us human.

Dr Leslie Weatherhead, one of the pioneers of the modern search for healing through psychology and religion, defines healing as 'the process of restoring the broken harmony which prevents personality, at any point of the body, mind or spirit, from its perfect functioning in its relevant environment: the body in the natural world; the mind in the realm of true ideas and the spirit in its relation with God.'[8]

This fundamental conception of health as synonymous with wholeness is taught consistently through Scripture and is illustrated in a number of ways. For example, Matthew 22:37, 39 'Love the Lord your God with all your *heart* and with all your *soul* and with all your *mind* . . . Love your *neighbour* as yourself.' Whether the New Testament is talking of coming to know God (1 Pet 2:24), worship (Mk 7:6), the body of Christ (1 Cor 12:12) or conduct (Jas 2:17) you will notice a common concern for integration and wholeness, for a balanced, unified working together of mind, body, emotions and relationships.

Individuation—authenticity and the creative life

As creatures of God's creation, in him we move and have our being. We are not our own. Health is very much dependent upon our acknowledging and responding to this fact with our whole being. As we have seen, Christ's saving and redeeming purpose was essentially to restore and affirm this fact. As creatures of God, we are uniquely shaped, and the only form or pattern of life this shape can comfortably and healthily fit is that of God. That is true both collectively and individually. Realising our own individual 'shape', our unique creation, is vital to health and wholeness. 'What we are, is God's gift to us. What we become, is our gift to him.'

Every person is a unique being unlike any other that existed before or will ever exist again. Every person born into this world represents something new. Deep inside each one of us is an energising and motivating psychic force, a sort of basic blueprint to be; within each one of us there is an inner centre that knows instinctively what constitutes health and well-being.

It is both our privilege and responsibility to realise and become what God has created us to be. Each one of us has to seek and discover his inner centre in order that an authentic person may begin to emerge, and that each individual 'truth' may be fully realised. Carl Jung called this movement towards one's inner self, 'individuation': individuation is the process that moves one to become a complete, unique person, and is vital to true health. To discover this uniqueness and maintain it is the challenge facing every human being.

> We either become what we are meant to be or are a caricature of our true self, an incomplete, distorted version of what was to be our true identity. Everything in nature seeks to realise itself and that is what individuation is all about.[9]

A creative life not realised becomes poisoned. Nature, when thwarted, takes her own revenge. This is a clear and undeniable fact, strongly supported by research. Much disease is caused, quite simply and fundamentally, by our failure to be honest and truthful — to ourselves, to each other and to the Creator. Deceit, expressed in all sorts of ways, mentally, emotionally, physically and socially, is at the root of so much dis-ease, and an acknowledgement of the fact is important to healing.

> To stay 'healthy' and fully alive it is essential to keep in touch with oneself. There is always a choice between avoiding truth by wearing a mask, and being authentic and facing reality. Remaining in touch with one's true self is the first requirement for continuing personal growth. 'The lie' brings violence and disorder into our natural self. It divides us against ourselves, alienates us from ourselves, makes enemies of ourselves and of the truth that is within us.[10]

> Every dishonest act is an act of self-denial. In that moment we cease to be. Only by being and saying what is really believed and felt does the individual participate in reality in a fundamental healthy sense.[11]

> Paradoxically, behind most, if not all illusions, is the desire for truth and freedom. Desperation frequently leads to illusions. The desperate person creates illusions to sustain his spirit in his struggle for survival. But the danger of an illusion is that it perpetuates the desperate condition. The more illusion rejects reality the more desperate becomes the struggle to support it.[12]

Individuation, of course, as will have been seen from our earlier discussion into the nature of man as a creature of God, is not an activity that springs from and focuses exclusively on man himself—though some secular philosophies and psychologies would have us believe this. We are not our own. God created us, and since we are a part of God's creation we are subject to the laws of that creation. We are nothing without him. The origin and goal of all human be-ing, then, is God. And the secret of our identity is hidden in the love and mercy of God. Our vocation is to work with God in the creation of our own life, our own identity, our own destiny. In this there is freedom and restraint. We actively participate in his creative freedom by choosing truth.

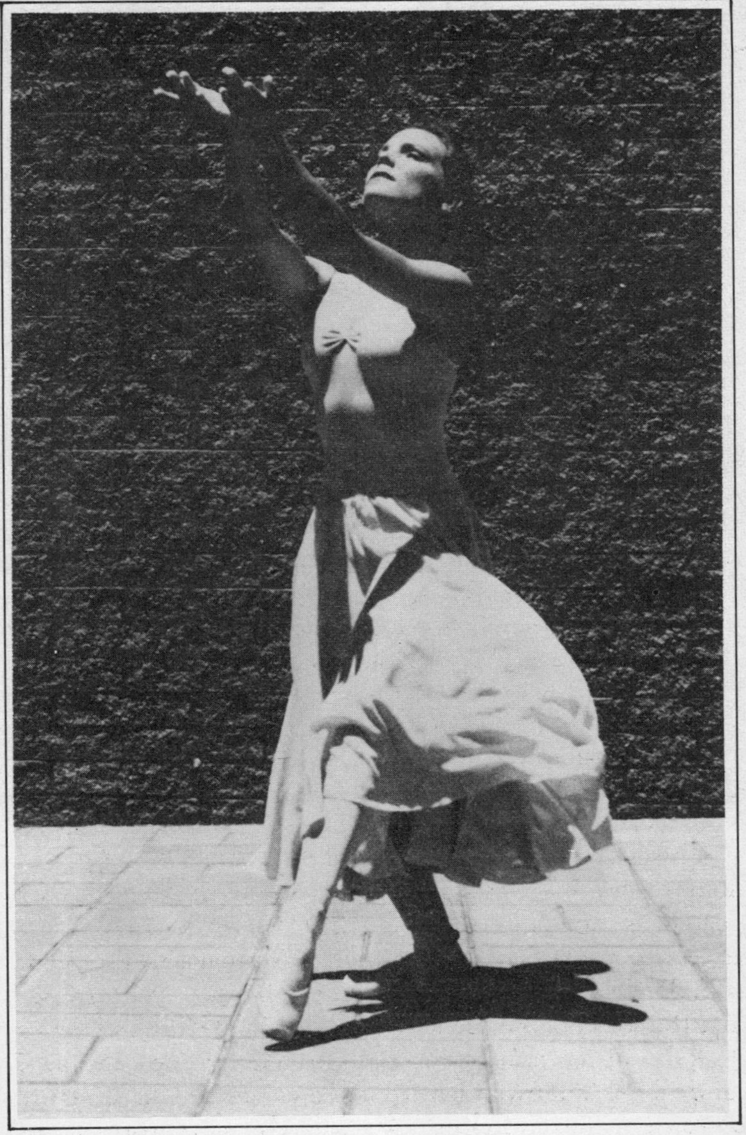

'Jesus, Son of David, have mercy on me!' (Mk 10:47).

To put it better, we are even called to share with God in the work of creating the truth of our identity. We can evade this responsibility by playing masks, and this pleases us because it can appear at times to be a free and creative way of living. But in the long run the cost and the sorrow come very high. To work at our own identity in God, which the Bible calls 'working' out our identity in God, is a labour that requires sacrifice and anguish, risk and many tears. It demands close attention to reality at every moment, and great fidelity to God as He reveals Himself, obscure in the mystery of each new situation.[13]

The way of peace is the way of truth. And truth, as we have already indicated, can be painful. Individuation and authenticity, essential to wholeness and well-being, can be very painful. Suffering and creativity, as any artist will vouch, go mysteriously together. To be a creator, as each one of us *is* with regard to his unique creature being, is almost synonymous with suffering. A commitment to *truth*, to authenticity and individuation as it relates to ourself, and the cross, is a commitment to suffer one's own 'death' in order to be reborn.

The proper good of a creature is to surrender itself to its Creator — to enact intellectually, volitionally, and emotionally, that relationship which is given in the mere fact of its being a creature. When it does so, it is happy. . . . In the world as we now know it, the problem is how to recover this self-surrender. We are not merely imperfect creatures who must be improved: we are, as Newman said, 'rebels who must lay down our arms'.[14]

'The root of dis-ease,' writes Frank Watts, 'is SIN: the word 'SIN' itself reveals the fundamental problem. At its centre is 'I' and we notice that 'I' is at the centre of prIde, guIlt and anxIety also!'[15] To be reborn is not easy! It is sometimes very painful. Individuation requires learning much about ourselves we would prefer not to know and assuming the burden of our inner conflicts:

> Growth is the dis-integration of one way of experiencing the world, followed by a re-organisation of this experience — a re-organising that includes new disclosures of the world. This organising, or even shattering, of one way to experience the world is brought on by new disclosures.[16]

On a more positive and encouraging note, according to Scripture not infrequently our dis-ease, arising out of deceit — psychological, sociological and physiological — can be an invitation to become authentic and whole. 'Pain,' writes C S Lewis, 'sometimes operates to shatter our man made illusions!'[17]

Individuation requires a submissive, faithful openness and honesty, a humility, a willingness to 'let go' and open oneself up, to make oneself vulnerable — to God, oneself and others — in order to be. There are, of course, all sorts of reasons and excuses why we find it difficult to let go. Some we have already identified. Others include fear, shame, guilt, ignorance, 'sickness', weakness, pride and arrogance. But no feeling of inadequacy, sense of fear or whatever can be accepted as an excuse not to come to Christ, since 'God did not send his Son into the world to condemn the world, but to save the world through him' (Jn 3:17) and give us health and wholeness.

So, as we are told in Hebrews 10:22 — 'Let us draw near to God with a sincere heart in full assurance of faith, having our hearts sprinkled to cleanse us from a guilty conscience and having our bodies washed with pure water.' And let us claim his promises in Scripture, asking in faith to be made authentic and whole.

Notes

1. P L Garlick, *Man's Search for Health* (Highway Press, 1952)
2. Morton Kelsey, *Healing and Christianity* (Harper and Row: London).
3. See C L Allen, *God's Psychiatry* (Power Books: Old Tappan, NJ) and H C Link, *None of These Diseases* (Lakeland: Basingstoke).
4. Jock Anderson, *Worship the Lord* (Inter-Varsity Press: Leicester, 1980).
5. Selwyn Hughes, *God Wants You Whole* (Kingsway: Eastbourne, 1984).
6. *Ibid*.
7. J P Baker, *Salvation and Wholeness* (Paulist Press).
8. B T Brown, *The Healing Ministry of the Church* (JBCE: Melbourne, 1986).
9. J A Sandford, *Healing and Wholeness* (Paulist Press).
10. Thomas Merton, *Conjectures of a Bystander* (Doubleday Image: London, 1968).
11. Clarke Moustakas, *Creative Life* (Van Nostrand Reinhold, 1977).
12. Alexander Lowen, *Betrayal of the Body* (Collier Macmillan: West Drayton, 1969).
13. Thomas Merton, *Seeds of Contemplation* (A Clarke: Wheathampstead, 1972).
14. C S Lewis, *The Problem of Pain* (Fontana: London).
15. Frank Watts, *Make All Things New*.
16. S M Jourad quoted in Otto and Mann *Ways of Growth* (Viking: London).
17. C S Lewis, *op. cit*.

2

Health and Healing Through Dance

Having identified the scriptural basis for health and healing, I now propose to look back to the origins of the understanding of dance as a means to health and healing.

Social, historical and anthropological roots of dance as therapy

The notion of dance as therapy is by no means a recent phenomenon. Contemporary interest is essentially a renewed interest, a rediscovery, in fact, of one of the oldest and most ancient of man's expressive forms which goes back to the very beginnings of civilisation. Dance, in all its many and varied forms and functions, has always played an important part in man's individual and collective human be-ing. Studies within sociology, history and anthropology across the continents, nations and cultures, which include evidence found in writings, artifacts, pictograms, etchings and drawings, as well as existing customs and traditions of primary societies, strongly testify to this fact.

Primitive man, especially, has always made use of this basic and holistic form of expression to 'speak' about the things important to himself and the community, things related to everyday life. Significantly, for primitive man

33

there was no distinction between life and dance. Dance was an expression of life in all its aspects. For the primitive man, also, everyday life was not divorced from religion. There was no distinction, as there is in our society today, between religious dance and other forms of dance. Dance, as with life, was religious. 'For the primitive man and society dance was never superficial or without purpose. It was not done because it was the thing to do, but because it was the thing.'[1] E Rosen writes:

> From the earliest times dancing was used in both natural and supernatural ways for the attainment of the most important ends of the community. In dance primitive man expressed everything that was life. There was little or no place for dance separate from life. He danced for joy, for grief and pain, for births, marriages, deaths, the crops, rain, the sun etc. etc. He danced everything that affected him emotionally and that could not be expressed in words — his fears, reverence, anxiety and awe. Physical movement with music and drama became the primary individual and collective means of expression and externalisation of thought. Through movement he communicated his deepest desires and convictions.[2]

'To this day,' writes R Katy, 'the primitive tribesmen of the Kalahari desert include everyone in the healing dance, and in the dance no distinction is made between physical, emotional and spiritual needs. The healing energy comes from the gods, and the dances and songs use this energy to facilitate the healing process.'[3]

R Alejandro, in describing the traditional dance of the Philippines writes:

> As with other primitive cultures, dance is used as a form of worship, as a framework for courtship or mating, as a way of expressing and reinforcing tribal unity and strength, and as a therapeutic or healing measure. Having both a religious and a social function the dance is used to appease the Gods; to solicit

rain; to seek deliverance from pestilence; to mark weddings, births, deaths and funerals; to prepare for war and combat; to celebrate victories.[4]

Kurt Sachs, writing about primitive dance says:

> The dance breaks down the distinctions of the body and soul, of abandoned expression of the emotions and controlled behaviour, of social life and the expression of isolation, of play, of religion and battle. In the ecstasy of dance man bridges the chasm between this and the other world, to the realm of spirits, demons and Gods. The dance has become the sacrificial rite, a charm, a prayer, a prophetic vision. It commands and dispels the forces of nature, heals the sick, links the dead to the chain of descendants. It assures the sustenance, luck of the chase, victory in battle, it blesses the field and the tribe.[5]

We see something of this primitiveness in the Old Testament. For the Jew then, as in some cases even today in Israel, there was no distinction between religious dance and other forms of dance. Dance was by definition, religious, and as such embraced every aspect of life, including personal and community health and healing.[6]

The idea, then, that dance can contribute to man's whole being — mental, physical, emotional, social and spiritual — is central to the lives of so-called primitive peoples throughout the world and its importance can hardly be over-estimated. This is of considerable significance for the purpose of this study. Dance is essentially primitive; it is a primary expression of human being. The instrument of expression, the vocabulary of expression and the expresser are one, all are integrated into a whole, concerned with life as a whole. In this sense of the term 'primitive', dance of the past is no different from dance of the present, dance as therapy.

The vigorous dancing so often displayed by primitive societies, which contributes, we are told, so effectively to working out physical and emotional tensions, encouraging enjoyable and valuable physical exercise, inducing profound mental and physical relaxation and providing an outlet for the expression of the self as well as binding together the participants — is no different in purpose and effect to ball-room dance, folk dance, disco and aerobic dance of today. All are equally 'primitive'.

For one of the best books intended as an introduction to the problems of dance in the context of human culture, and for a fuller discussion of the role which dance has played throughout the different stages of evolution of the human race I recommend *The Nature of Dance — an anthropological perspective* by R Lange (Macdonald and Evans: Plymouth, 1975). Lange argues that the appreciation of dance as a human faculty has long been neglected as it has been dominated by an almost exclusive conception of dance as 'high art', dance as 'aesthetic contemplation' and passive entertainment:

> My personal approach to dance has been fundamentally changed after spending twelve years in research. All my previous ideas on dance, its relationship to human being and its history, collapsed, when they were confronted by the facts of dance met in remote villages throughout the world. One has to bow to the human dignity still preserved in the old patterns of life, where dance has always played a vital role in organising the whole of life. Man, although he creates his culture, does not cease to be a biological being. Man, being a unique species, has to act in his own special way, but at the same time according to the laws of biological makeup. As soon as this is brought out of balance, disturbed human beings are the result.

Lange is speaking as a social anthropologist, and is focusing on the biological nature of man, but he is bringing out the principle that we have already identified from the Scriptures. Man is not his own. He is subject to laws — God-given, natural laws — and when these laws are broken or not met, then he can expect dis-ease. Lange goes on to list some of the many and varied functions of dance. Significantly, these include relieving emotional tension, releasing surplus energy, releasing physical discomfort, reinforcing social patterns and values, encouraging community, sexual sublimation, exercise, religious ritual, and non-verbal language of expression. He concludes:

> It therefore becomes evident that knowledge of the biological [sociological, psychological and philosophical] aspect of dance not only has significance as yet another element in the historical perspective of human development but indeed, it has great contemporary value that still has not been explored and appreciated enough. The biological [sociological, psychological and philosophical] aspect of dance has an educational, recreational and rehabilitative relevance . . . these dance manifestations . . . may not belong to art, they may not be included in the investigations led by aestheticians (or the arts council!) but nevertheless they are an essential part of human development.

Dance, I believe, *is* a seriously neglected and underestimated part of man's human being. It *is* one of the few truly holistic activities involving, as it does, the mind, body, emotions and community. It *is* one of the truly authentic experiences, potentially at least, in that the dance and the dancer are both the form and the content of experience and expression. As Martha Graham noted, 'Dance, of all languages tells the truth.' Truth, as we shall see later on, is a prerequisite of all health and healing. I strongly believe, along with Lange, that there is a serious need to redefine dance within Western society today, to rediscover and restore it to its more primary state as a means of communal and individual well-being. Are the values and justifications of primitive dance so alien, so inappropriate, to today's society? I think not. It may be that the forms of expression and the context in which dance is expressed have both changed, but man has not changed. The needs and drives of primitive man are the primitive needs and drives of all men, in all places, and at all times.

I am reminded of a very interesting piece of dance research carried out by the sociologist Frances Rust in the sixties. She set out to identify some of the values related to social dance among adolescents in polytechnics and colleges of further education. Significantly, her findings are dominated precisely by those values and justifications which characterise primitive dance, and go a long way to testifying to those 'most original and enduring fundamentals'. It is clear that the justifications as expressed by these teenagers of the sixties at least, are no different from the descriptions and justifications of primitive societies. I list just some of these findings. We shall be referring to this justification in more detail in Part 2 under 'The Social Dimension of Human Being'.

Polytechnic students' attitudes
Girls' reasons for liking 'beat'
Escape valve to get rid of pent-up emotions
An outlet for emotions
Can pour all my energy and tension out
Helps relieve tension
Physical exercise but also mentally relaxing
Induces a spirit of enjoyment and happiness and makes people
    relax
Can let my hair down; experiment, exhibit; lose inhibitions
Vibrant
Can let myself go
The fun, the rhythm, the excitement
Gets people in the right mood at a party
Simply enjoy dancing
Easy to do
No tedious lessons; almost anyone can do them
No stereotype footwork; flexibility of movements
Nobody notices if you cannot dance

Can express feelings which the music stimulates
Expressive
Gives you a chance to express yourself in movement
Free expression of how you feel at the moment
It exercises the whole body
Strong quick and exciting movements
A chance to loosen my limbs
Movements natural and stimulated by a lively beat
Form of display to the opposite sex
Physical stimulation
Because of the sexual undertones
Can meet the opposite sex in an informal way
Useful for meeting girls of my own age
Opportunity to meet friends
The atmosphere—very informal

College of high education—full-time business studies
Boys' attitudes to 'beat'
It's good fun and I enjoy it
I enjoy the sensationalism
It allows me to go mad to a limited extent and to let off
    steam in a fairly safe way
It gives me a chance to work off excess energy
They give me a way of expressing feelings in action, and
    letting off steam
You let off pent up emotions and meet the best of females
They are lively and usually put you in a happy mood
It gets your feelings out of your system and it's stimulating
It's great fun
Because of the rhythm
It stimulates my emotions to the opposite sex
They are stimulating
Sexy; intimate
I like seeing girls' bosoms bounce
I can dance how I like
More freedom and more movement to dance
They are informal and easy and uninhibited
Complete freedom of style and speed

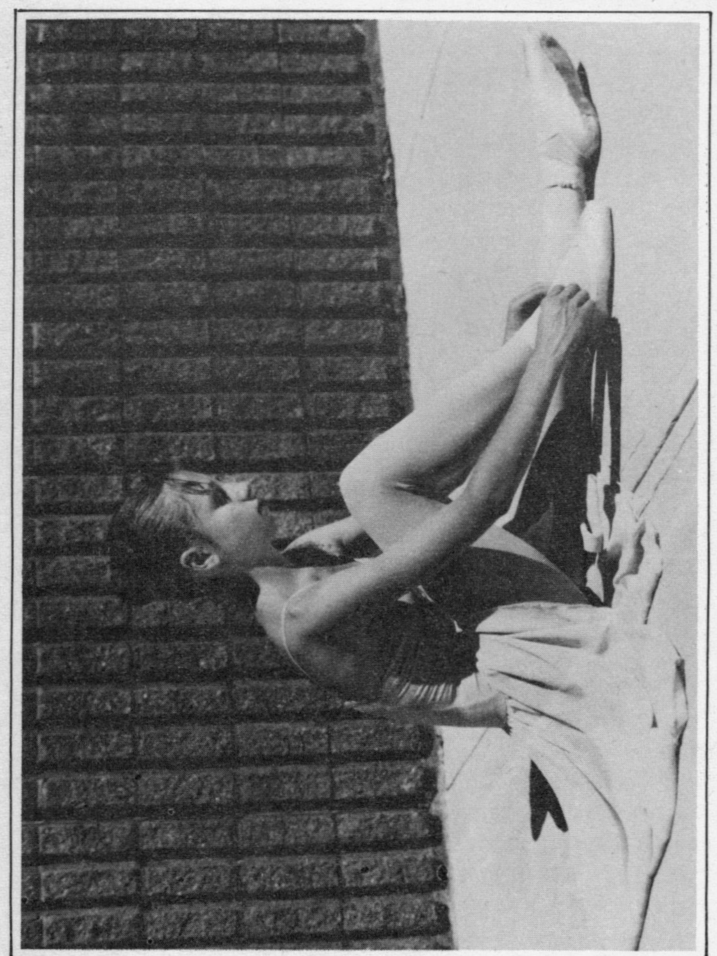

'In quietness and trust is your strength' (Is 30:15).

Other reasons from other groups:
You can dance on your own or in a crowd and when you feel like
    it and not have to be asked — and start and stop as you please
You do not need a partner; a group of girls can do it together
Anyone can have a 'go'; everyone can join in
You can create your own variations without being tied to
    someone else
You can express how you feel when you dance modern
Enjoyment: gives me a kick
You can let yourself go — nobody really cares what they look
    like to other people watching
If without a girl friend you can still dance by yourself or with
    a crowd of boys
It is not so much the beat dances that I enjoy but the
    atmosphere, girls and music that you get in these places[7]

As R Lange poignantly remarks, 'These justifications may not belong to art, they may not be included in investigations led by aestheticians or arts counsellors, but, nevertheless, they are an essential part of human development.'[8]

Early twentieth century modern dance

The beginning of the twentieth century witnessed something of a revolution in Western dance, and the approach to dance as therapy and wholeness has, in part at least, grown directly out of that revolution. As we shall see, many of the values underlying the thoughts and actions of these early dance pioneers are essentially those of dance therapy.

Early twentieth century modern dance, with its intense desire to express the totality of human being through movement — especially natural and spontaneous movement, with its concern for psychological, sociological and physical openness and honesty, for authenticity and truth, for seeking new and freer, more authentic and appropriate ways of expression, is very much a part of today's dance as therapy. Its rebellious philosophy; its deliberate and emphatic breaking with what was regarded as fading and élitist art concepts, frozen modes of expression, rigid stylised conformity, high manners—and, towards the end of the nineteenth century, not so high manners; its emphasis on theatricalism, formal structures, romantic idealism and illusion; its concern with the superhuman, supernatural and super spiritual; and, above all, its passionate concern to restore dance to its rightful place among the people, for the people, representing the needs and interests of ordinary people—all these are very much a part of dance therapy as we know it today.

Writings of the early twentieth century dance pioneers

My concern with looking at some of the dance innovators of the early twentieth century is not so much to identify their contribution to theatrical dance, important as that is, but to identify something of their philosophy of life and their view of dance and its relationship to life, both individual and communal. If there is one thing that distinguishes the early modern dancers from contemporary modern dancers it is this commitment first of all to life, rather than dance for its own sake. In their thinking, as well as their dancing, there is a passionate and compassionate commitment to the authentic life of both the individual and the community. Frequently, as we shall see, their thinking was rooted in a profound religious belief—something totally alien to today's dance! Many of the early pioneers in modern dance were, in fact, explicitly religious. In the 1930s Ruth St Dennis founded 'The Society of Spiritual Arts' at the Church of Divine Dance. Ted Shawn, her one-time famous partner, was a theological student. Doris Humphrey's work is frequently implicitly religious, for example, *Passacaglia*.

Let us look at some of the writings of these pioneers.

ISADORA DUNCAN

If we seek the real source of the dance, if we go to nature, we find that the dance of the future is the dance of the past, the dance of eternity, and has been and will always be the same . . . the movements of the savage, who lived in freedom, in constant touch with nature, were unrestricted natural and beautiful. Only the movements of the naked body can be perfectly natural. Man, arriving at the end of civilisation, will have to return to nakedness, not to the unconscious nakedness of the savage, but the consciousness of the mature Man, whose body will be the harmonious expression of his spiritual being.

Dance is the highest expression in the freest body.[9]

LOUIS FULLER

Surprise, deception, contentment, uncertainty, resignation, hope, distress, joy, fatigue, feebleness, and finally death. Are not all these sensations, each one in turn, the lot of humanity? And why cannot these things be expressed by the dance, guided intelligently, as well as by life itself?

Motion has been the starting point of all effort at self expression and it is faithful to nature.[10]

RUTH ST DENNIS

Dancing as a life experience is not something to be taken from the outside — something painfully to be learned or something to be imitated. Dancing is the natural, rhythmic movement of the body that has long been suppressed or distorted, and to dance would have been as natural as to eat, or to run, or swim, if our civilisation had not in countless ways and for diverse reasons put its ban upon this instinctive and joyous action of the harmonious being. Our formal religions, our crowded cities, our clothes and our transportation are all largely responsible for the inert mass of humanity.

Let us regard dance fundamentally as a life experience, as

the primitive and ultimate means of self expression and communication. Let us see in the free, spontaneous dance of every child the beginning of the universal language and the universal art which, largely unconscious to itself, grows bodily into words, telling of illusive and exquisite moments of the hidden self.[11]

MARY WIGMAN

The dance is one of many human experiences which cannot be suppressed. Dancing has existed at all times, and among all people and races.

Dance . . . presupposes a heightened, increased life response. Moreover, the heightened response does not always have to have a happy background. Sorrow, pain, even horror and fear, tend also to release a welling-up feeling, and therefore set free the dancer's whole being.[12]

MARTHA GRAHAM

Throughout time dance has not changed in one essential function. The function of the dance is communication. The responsibility to see that dance fulfills its function belongs to us who are dancing today as it did to those of yesterday.[13]

JOSE LIMON

The dance is all things to all men. Parents are delighted and amazed at the instinctive response of their infant to music, 'Look, he's dancing.' Children do not walk to school, or into the dining room, or upstairs to bed. The adolescent is notorious for his nervous, jittery dances. And love's young dream: imagine our early romances without a waltz by moonlight! We discover the rapture and intoxication of love during dance. And even maturity finds a new dimension to the eery business of existence during the sedate ritual of ballroom: a suspension, a surcease, an inexplicable lifting of the spirit, when even the corns cease to hurt. The dance is an activism.

It has been with us since we became humans, and no doubt before that. It will be with us to the end. It is a human necessity, profound, and not to be denied. Puritans have banned and proscribed it at various times as the work of the devil, happily without success. I believe that we are never more truly and profoundly human than when we dance.[14]

MARGARET N H DOUBLER

Dance education must be emotional, intellectual and spiritual, as well as physical, if dance is to contribute to the larger aims of education... the development of personality through conscious experience... Of all the arts, dance is peculiarly suited to such a fulfilment of the personality. It serves all the ends of the individual growth: it helps to develop the body; it stimulates the imagination and challenges the intellect; it helps to cultivate an appreciation of beauty and it opens and refines the emotional nature.[15]

VIRGINIA STEWART

The modern dance springs out of the very heart of man. It goes back to the source of human life. It throws away superficiality and moves out into the open spaces where abide the heart and soul of mankind. In its marvellous harmony of oneness with the great things of nature, the body and soul come into a unity with the cosmos.[16]

ARTHUR MICHEL

Where the ballet had denied reality, modern dance affirmed it. The aim of the latter was to create from *life*, not from technique. The experiences of the realities of life in their deepest and most intensive forms, from the direct to the mystic, ecstatic conquests of metaphysics.

These artists have given us something priceless. They have restored the dance to its ancient function, and proven to the modern world that it can reveal, instruct and ennoble. It can exult. It can ritualise the great tragedies and ecstasies of man. It is in the power and province of dance to reaffirm the dignity of man in an age that desperately needs this affirmation. Never have the arts been so much needed, nor so challenged, as in these times of mechanised bestiality, when the human species seems possessed by a suicidal frenzy. Surely the dance can remind us of the greatness of man's spirit, and of his creativeness, not his destructiveness. The dance is many things. It is power. It can help stem the putrefaction and decay gnawing at the heart of human courage, and withstand the philosophy of doom and surrender. The dancer can use his voice to call for reason out of unreason, and order out of disorder. That has always been the high task of the artist.[17]

Here, then, we have a marvellous glimpse of just a few of the pioneers of modern dance. What extraordinarily articulate and visionary people they were! I strongly recommend further reading of recent dance history.[18]

There appear to be some common threads running through all these writings and it might be helpful to identify these by way of summarising some of the contributions made by pioneers to dance therapy.

First, they were all 'giants': extraordinarily committed people, committed not just to dance, but to life itself. Underlying all their thinking is a profound commitment to life and to living. Dance, as with primitive societies, was not separate from life, but was intimately related to life.

Secondly, they had a genuine commitment to truth, to open, natural honesty. This is expressed not just in their writings and their dancing but in every aspect of their life.

Thirdly, authenticity in self-expression is a priority. Original, creative self-expression is the key to modern dance.

Fourthly, all shared a deep commitment to the therapeutic and educational powers of dance. They all believed in the integrative, healing and restoring potential of dance for the mind, body, emotions, community and spirit.

Fifthly, they all sought to express these new-found truths in a relevant way. Theirs was a commitment to communication—to all people rather than an exclusive minority. They believed that dance belonged to all people and that it was a natural and essential expression of all.

Where have all these visionaries of dance gone? Where are the dance 'giants' of today? Are the values and justifications for dance as expressed in the writings of these pioneers so alien, so irrelevant and so inappropriate to contemporary society? How do you see your place as a dancer, especially as a Christian dancer, in the life of human being today?

Dance and community today

As we have looked at twentieth-century and primitive dance we have seen a conception of dance very different from, if not totally alien to that which characterises dance today, with its ever-increasing 'functional exclusiveness' as an economic, 'high art' enterprise, performed by a minority and élite group of *professionals* to only a minority and élite audience. The notion of multifunctional dance, and dance for the community as a whole, seems very far from the minds of institutions and those whose concern it is to develop dance in society today. And yet never has the time been so appropriate for such an expansion. Western society today is undergoing an economic and social revolution, and for the first time in our history society as a whole, rather than a small aristocratic élite, is being forced to consider the problem of having time on its hands. It may be that in the not-so-distant future life will no longer be dominated exclusively by the need to work.

> There is ample evidence that recreation and leisure represent increasingly a major element in human life. Giving attention to understanding this phenomenon is in no sense a frivolous activity and must receive the investment of able scientists of many disciplines and theoretical persuasions.[19]

In view of the increase in leisure time and decrease in work time, the ever-increasing life expectancy, the growing enlightenment with regard to holistic health and overall individual and social well-being, it is not possible to justify the present highly exclusive and narrow conception of dance.

As someone who has for the past twenty years been partly responsible for preparing dancers and dance teachers, I am particularly conscious of the narrow and élitist approach to dance that is the result of our dance education. While I recognise a genuine attempt on the part of some dance institutions to correct this weakness, I have reluctantly to admit that in the main it results in little more than lip service, simply because so very few opportunities exist for community dance, or any dance other than entertainment, and anyway the ambition of a majority of students is to be in a 'proper' dance company! Most dance students have as their ideal what is essentially a reinforcement of the status quo.

Dance, it has to be admitted, is a marginal art. For most people it has little or no relevance to their daily lives. To create anything that has relevance outside the very narrow limits of the traditional dance world, a dancer has to make the connection between dance *and* everyday life. Until I did that I could not accept the image of myself as a dancer.[20]

Long ago the person and the artist were inseparable. They lived in a world which demanded constant participation. The hunters learnt to use song and dance as a medium to approach the gods. Their painted bodies and masks contained the spirit of the animals they hunted. They were our first artists. They expressed their attitudes to life, their experiences, joy and pain through body and voice...we are all artists. We all possess creative potential. It is present at birth and it disappears at death. But for too many, it remains latent and unrecognised. The worst evil is that we have accorded hands-off status to the few who have recognised, developed and marketed this instinct in themselves. We tip our hats and whisper ARTIST! from the grey sidelines. When they pass the million-dollar mark in the performance arts we breath STAR![21]

The removal of art from life, the divorce of aesthetic and ethical decisions from the mundane has reached its zenith. Artistic masterpieces have seldom been part of the everyday loves of everyday people. We are a society which has given over the keeping of our aesthetic judgements to professionals, museums, art historians and critics. We go to visit actual works of art in museums (and dance theatres) almost as an act of homage.[22]

In speaking about the need to restore the arts to the wider society of everyday people, living everyday lives, Chris Johnson writes:

The aim is to touch those things deep within all communities — the sense of festival, religious rite, ritual. It's all part of the attempt to bring art out of the concert hall and gallery (as well as the opera houses and dance theatres) onto the streets and back into everyday life, to shrug off the general anaestheia induced by technology, to actively create our culture rather than passively receive it.[23]

It should be clear that my concept of dance is multifunctional and multidimensional. It is concerned with 'wholeness' in the broadest sense of the term and with life in all its manifestations. My concern is not with any particular aesthetic form in the sense of classical ballet, ballroom, tap, modern, jazz, disco, historic, national, ethnic, folk etc, all of which have their own distinct style, movement vocabulary, structures, forms and intentions. My concept of dance as therapy is an 'umbrella' one, embracing a wide variety of expressions, forms, functions and meanings. All have a legitimate place in so far as they contribute to man's wholeness and well-being.

There is no one distinct and definite form to denote 'therapeutic dance'. In the sense that all dance forms can directly or indirectly contribute to health and healing, all are potentially therapeutic.

Common to all dance forms are the following:
(1) All use the human body as their instrument of expression.
(2) All use movement as their means of expression.
(3) All recognise the non-verbal nature of their expression. All, whatever their motivations and structure, have this one basic thing in common.

Medicine: medical and social science

The third main source for dance as therapy comes from medicine: medical and social science.

One of the compulsory readings as an undergraduate in the social sciences of the sixties was an article by Becker entitled 'Whose Side Am I On?' In it Becker argues that the sort of scientific certainty and objectivity for which social scientists are seeking constitutes, in fact, a 'categorical mistake', in that it attempts to apply the canons, logic and truth of one paradigm, namely science and mathematics, to that of an essentially different paradigm, human sciences. He argues that the physical science paradigm is inappropriate when it comes to the uniqueness and complexity of human behaviour. In seeking objectivity and truth the best one can possibly hope for is a disciplined concern to indentify and understand one's personal subjectivities. The concept of 'paradigm' was developed by Kuhn who used the term originally to describe the set of assumptions held by a particular community of scientific scholars in a specific historic era. Paradigm refers not only to the corpus of knowledge which constitutes a subject or discipline but also to the belief about research procedures, key problems, and how they might be solved. A paradigm describes and explains a specific set of canons of logic and truth, and a particular conception of reality.

What has all this to do with dance as therapy? First, as dance therapists we need to ask ourselves whose side we are on. That is, what assumptions, biases, logic, and value orientations underlie our notion of dance, human being, health and healing. More often than not these fundamental attitudes are taken for granted and rarely identified. More often than not the dancer works intuitively and unconsciously, if not without concern about such questions. But it is important to recognise and understand the paradigms within dance therapy and to know where one stands. The disciplines of psychology and sociology, like dance, cover a wide variety of forms and expressions about the nature and conditions of man and society. No one paradigm has monopoly of the truth! All in their different ways contribute to making sense of human being. Social psychology is a vast and complex field with its own paradigms.

It is not my purpose to involve the reader in too detailed a discussion of the significance of the differences between various schools of thought, but it is important in such a study as this that the reader is made aware of such fundamental differences. The question that is of crucial importance to the Christian healer is, 'How do these different schools of social psychology relate to the Bible?' As a *Christian* 'healer' what are your basic assumptions about the nature and condition of man and society? How do they affect your ministry of health and healing?

There are three major streams of thought within the disciplines of social psychology. The first two are well known and well established: psychoanalysis and behaviourism. The third is perhaps less well known. It is sometimes referred to as 'the third force', because it is seen as an alternative to the traditional approaches to health and healing. But more generally it is known by the title 'Humanistic Psychology' (not to be confused with humanism).

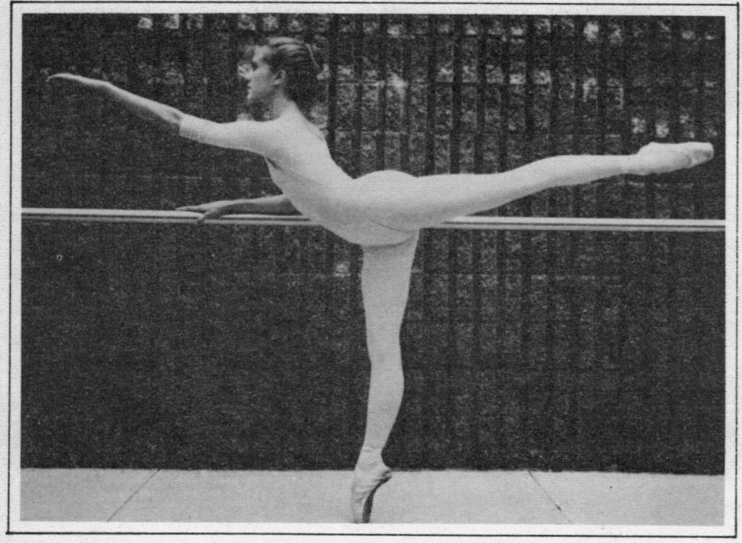

'We are temples of God (2 Cor 7:1). *Let us honour God with our bodies* (1 Cor 6:19), *purifying ourselves from everything that contaminates it, perfecting holiness out of our reverence for God'* (2 Cor 7:1).

Expressive arts therapies lie mainly within this third force. The reasons for this are by no means clear cut or in any sense universal, but in the main the various 'schools' which go to make up this third force are characteristically much more open, less rigid, more varied and experimental. They are not reductionist in their approach and all have a primary concern for the body and non-verbal behaviour in a way that the other two major psychologies, traditionally at least, do not. Hence dance therapy's relationship with this 'paradigm'. But this identification is relatively loose and, in the main, not formally established. This is inevitable, given the history and nature of dance therapy. Therapy is still in its infant stages and a clear, formalised philosophy, psychology and sociology of dance is still being worked out. Perhaps what is exciting, is the growing recognition of the need for such a formal base. This is a consistent theme of journals and articles within dance therapy.

For the Christian healer, however, there already exists a formal base from which he can reliably and validly work. But it should be understood that the Bible is not a medical treatise. While it has, in the God-given 'laws' already referred to, all the principles of health and healing that we need, it remains man's responsibility and obligation to translate such principles into disciplined, public, everyday truths. This is particularly so for the dancer who intends therapy to be a full-time ministry, and wishes to make it a reliable and credible professional force within both the church and community.

As indicated, for the most part dance therapy identifies with Humanistic Psychology. Let us have a look for a moment at some of the writings of this school, and try to identify common characteristics as they relate to dance.

F Wells writes:

There is ample evidence to demonstrate that many therapists now seriously question, if they have not already abandoned, the traditional medical models, preferring the more humanistic view of seeing dis-ease more in terms of 'self-growth', 'self-improvement' and 'self-actualisation' than as treatment and disorder.

Incredible as it may seem, the dichotomy between mind and body still persists in the Western world. The view still prevails that the mind represents the cognitive and the rational and the body the emotional and irrational . . . and that verbal language is the expression of the former and the non-verbal of the latter. This view is still the traditional assumption in most psycho-therapies which flows from the conviction that none but verbal therapy can be useful in the treatment of mental and emotional disease.[24]

As E and B Feder put it,

The bulk of psychotherapy is overwhelmingly verbal and talk orientated, healing is by conversation. It rests on the implicit assumption that the psyche resides in the head and must be approached in the language of the heard word. The old distinctions between psyche and soma still prevail, for the most part, and the old hierarchies still rule. The relationship between mind and body is acknowledged in modern medium, but is almost always expressed as psychosomatic rather than somatopsychic.[25]

In terms of expressive arts therapy most psychologists are still sceptical of any but verbal methods of therapy. There is still suspicion that art therapies, body work, social work and diet and nutrition have little to do with improving the mental-emotional complex.

Talking out is still the only accepted form of work!

Recently, however, role play, psychodrama, sociodrama, music therapy, bioenergetics, dance therapy, megavitamin therapy, self-development groups, self-actualising groups, Gestalt and many more therapists of the humanistic school have entered the scene and have shown significantly that non-verbal therapy does have a reliable and credible place within therapy generally. Body and mind are interactive and the problem of dis-ease can be significantly influenced from either side, psyche or soma. When psychotherapy brings about a change in mental attitude, there should be a corresponding physical change. Similarly, when the dance therapist brings about a change in body behaviour, there should be a corresponding change in mind. This represents the essential basis of dance and movement therapy. Whereas the approach to verbal therapy is through 'mind-body', the approach of dance therapy is through 'body-mind.'

Arthur Janov points out that 'explanation talk', or 'about talk', which tends to predominate in conventional verbal therapy, has the effect of keeping feelings diluted. The 'explain your feelings' talk of many middle-class homes frequently blocks direct emotional expression and discharge.[26]

One of the weaknesses of exclusively verbal therapy is its tendency to ignore the physical/feeling dimensions of the individual's health and healing. It excludes almost totally the body derived felt level of experiencing; it fails to recognise that the felt level must precede the conceptual level of the person. He must not be cut off from his kinesthetic/affective reaction. Verbalisation often serves to alienate further the individual from his experimental body process since it causes one to adopt the role of an observer looking at one's self, rather than being the active participant creating one's own experience.[27]

An important leader within the area of body/feeling is Alexander Lowen, a psychiatrist who has developed a method called bioenergetics. 'It is the axiom of bioenergetic analysis that a person can only feel his body. One cannot feel the environment except through its effects upon the body. In reality, then, one feels how one's body reacts to the environment or to external objects, and perception of this feeling is projected upon the stimulus. All our feelings are body perceptions (conscious or unconscious). How much we feel and how deeply we feel is a function of self awareness.'

There is so close an interaction between the muscular sequence involved in all expressive movements and psychic attitude that not only does the psychic attitude connect up with the muscular states, but also every sequence of tension and relaxation provokes a specific attitude. When there is a specific motor sequence, it changes the inner situation and attitude.[28]

So dominated is traditional therapy by the rational, the analytic and objective that we seem to have lost contact with the less rational or non-rational and intuitive aspect of our being. Jungian analyst and dance therapist, Irene Champer-nouve, warns that:

> Verbalisation may distance the communication of the individual, by introducing an intermediate language with the attendant dangers of mistranslation and misinterpretation. It is much easier for an individual to conceal his feelings and thoughts in verbal communication than it is in movement. Unlike verbal language, the language of the body never ceases, even in response. It betrays our innermost thoughts. When words are removed we have more time to direct our thoughts to observing our own ongoing behaviour, as well as others. Individuals who have learned effective verbal defences, from silence to intellec-tualisation—and that includes most westerners—need new methods, new channels or avenues of response and communi-cating. Movement responses which involve a lower brain level are somehow less a part of conscious awareness and therefore sometimes more reliable expressions of feelings than words.

Altshuler points to the fact that the thalamus, which is the seat of all sensation, emotion and aesthetic feeling, is not involved in mental illness, and that patients who cannot be reached by verbal messages to the brain can be aroused by music by way of the thalamus, which when stimulated auto-matically relays the sensations to the brain.[29]

Jung's work has given special credence to the use of art, and by implication dance, as a means by which the uncon-scious can by-pass the more conscious, thus encouraging the patient to become more an object to himself. Jung viewed the artistic experience, what he called the 'active imagination', as having both a diagnostic and therapeutic function. The crea-tive act evokes material that is available for analysis and is at the same time cathartic. The cathartic function, common to all expressive therapies, is based upon the well-known and proven finding that the expression of a problem provides release and relief. By virtue of the non-literal or apparently non-rational — but *not* irrational — aspects of the creative act, deep and often unconscious feelings that defy words can be symbolically represented. Both conscious and unconscious material can be given form.

In 'Creative Dance and Therapy' Bender and Boas et al document support for Jung's position.[30] They found that the primary nature of spontaneous dance had within it the potential of stimulating and giving expression to primitive unconscious as well as helping the 'dancers' to deal with their conflicts through the creative act. Similarly, Mary Whitehouse, a dance therapist in California, speaks of the flow of unconscious material coming out in physical form.[31]

> In creative and artistic pursuits the dis-eased person can give aesthetic form to deep-lying wishes, fears and conflicts. The essential qualities which result from these activities, the fun, excitement, escape, the pleasurable sensations, the inner feelings of fulfillment . . . all serve to relieve tension and anxiety.[32]

Since tension is invariably both mental and physical, a basic principle of dance therapy is that relief in one aspect will mean relief in the other.

Modern dance uses the same primitive elements which our early ancestors used, but employs them in a different way. Primitive man expressed in the most direct way possible — through rhythmic bodily movement — his reverential awe at the world of mystery and wonder about him; the modern dancer with less awe, perhaps, and a more intelligent sense of wonder expresses, as directly, his reaction to a more complex world.[33]

The task of the dance therapist is to create opportunities for people to move in new and satisfying ways, to rediscover their bodies, to get in touch with what goes on inside and find ways to express it 'outside' in order to bring the individual to a greater degree of unification through awareness of self.

Dance as an art form at the professional level achieves its most significant results through the work of its great artists and companies. Dance as education, as therapy, achieves its most significant results through the growth of the individual. The medium of both is movement. Both deal with dance as an art form, but an important difference exists in motivation and intention.

A summary and comparison model of traditional psychotherapy and humanistic psychotherapy

In order to help the reader become clearer about the distinguishing nature and conditions of humanistic psychology as opposed to psychoanalytic and behaviourist psychology—and therefore become clearer about the general nature of dance as therapy which I am proposing—it might be useful to list some of the important differences. It must be understood that these comparisons are gross oversimplifications. They are models and therefore do not represent reality: in order to help us, a model expresses complex reality in simplified terms.

Traditional medical model	*Contemporary humanistic model*
Concerned with sickness and disease	Concerned with self-actualisation
'Normative' non-problematic model	'Interpretive' problematic model
Functional	Humanist
Verbal emphasis	Non-verbal emphasis
Objectivity/analysis	Subjectivity/synthesis
Language orientated	Non-language orientated
Sickness orientated	Health orientated
Cognitive emphasis	Affective emphasis
Mind emphasis	Body emphasis
Particularistic	Holistic
Rational	Non-rational
Analytical	Intuitive
Theoretical/experimental	Phenomenological/observational

The 'Articles of Association' of the American Association of Humanistic Psychology defines the thrust of humanistic therapy as being

> primarily an orientation toward the whole of psychology rather than a distinct area or school. It stands to respect the worth of persons, respect for different approaches, open-mindedness as to acceptable methods, an interest in exploration of new aspects of human behaviour.
>
> As a 'third force' in contemporary psychology it is concerned with topics that have little place in existing theories and systems: love, creativity, self, growth organism, basic need gratifications, self activity, higher values, being, becoming, spontaneity, play, humour, affection, naturalness, warmth, egotranscendence, objectivity, autonomy, responsibility means, transcendental experience, courage and relative concepts.

Key phrases in humanistic health and healing are 'here and now', 'feeling rather than thinking'.

I am beginning to believe that we may be seeing dance come a full circle. Man originally danced not to entertain or make a living in high art, but to express himself and his community in ways that words could not, and should not, express. He danced for health, in the broadest sense of the term, he danced for the sheer joy of moving. When he danced he reflected his whole being and that of the community. Is it too much to hope that this may yet again be part of human being? As Mary Wigman said, 'I feel that the dance is a language which is inherent, but slumbering, in every one of us. It is possible for every human being to experience the dance as an expression of his own body, and in his own way'.[34]

> I see men and women dancing rhythmically in joy on a hill top bathed in the saffron rays of a setting sun. I see them moving slowly, with flowing, serene gestures, in the glow of the risen moon. I see them giving praise, praise for the earth and the sky and the sea and the hills, in free, happy movements that are

projections of their moods of peace and adoration. I see Dance being used as a means of communication between soul and soul — to express what is too deep, too fine for words.

The word Dancer should rightly mean one who expresses in bodily gesture the joy and power of his being.[35]

Notes

1. Walter Sorrell, *Dance throughout the Ages* (Crossett and Dunlop, 1967).
2. E Rosen, *Dance and Psychotherapy* (Dance Horizons, 1974).
. R Katy quoted in E and B Feder, *Expressive Arts Therapy* (Prentice-Hall: Hemel Hempstead).
4. R Alejandro, 'Dance in the Philippines', *Dancescope*.
5. Kurt Sachs, *World History of Dance*.
6. See Martin Blogg, *Dance and the Christian Faith* (Hodder and Stoughton: London, 1985).
7. Frances Rust, *Dance in Society* (Routledge and Kegan Paul: London).
8. R Lange, *The Nature of Dance* (MacDonald and Evans: Plymouth, 1975).
9. J M Brown Ed, *Visions of Modern Dance* (Dance Books: London).
10. *Ibid*.
11. *Ibid*.
12. *Ibid*.
13. *Ibid*.
14. *Ibid*.
15. *Dance: a Creative Experience* (University of Wisconsin Press).
16. Virginia Stewart and M Armitage, *The Modern Dance* (1970).
17. J M Brown Ed, *op cit*.
18. *Ibid*.
19. J R Kelly *Leisure* (Allen and Unwin: London).
20. Andy Solway, article in *New Internationalist*, no 144 (February, 1985).
21. Chris Sheppard, *ibid*.
22. Linda Cabe, *ibid*.
23. Chris Johnson, *ibid*.

24. F Wells quoted in W Anderson Ed, *Therapy and the Expressive Arts* (Harper and Row: London).
25. R Katy, *op cit*.
26. J Liss, *Freedom to Feel* (Wildwood House).
27. W Anderson Ed, *op cit*.
28. P Schilder quoted in Alexander Lowen Ed, *Betrayal of the Body* (Collier MacMillan: West Drayton, 1969).
29. Altshuler, 'Music Therapy Retrospective and Perspective', bulletin for the National Association of Music Therapists, (January, 1953).
30. Bender and Boas, 'Creative Dance and Therapy', *American Journal of Orthopsychiatry*, vol 11 no 41.
31. Mary Whitehouse, 'An Approach to the Centre', *Psychology Perspectives* (3 April, 1972).
32. E Rosen, *op cit*.
33. M Lloyd, *Borzio Book of Modern Dance* (Dance Horizons, 1949).
34. C J Cohen, *Dance as Theatre Art* (Dodd and Mead, 1974).
35. J M Brown Ed, *op cit*.

PART 2

Four Dimensions of Human Being

3

The Mental Dimension of Human Being

Scripture and mental health

Scripture has a great deal to say about the mind and mental well-being (see Ephesians 5, Galatians 5 and 6). It is clear that 'what' and 'how' we think largely determines the way we feel and the way we act. 'For as he thinks within himself, so he is' (Prov 23:7, NIV margin). 'The eye is the lamp of the body. If your eyes are good, your whole body will be full of light. But if your eyes are bad, your whole body will be full of darkness.' (Mt 6:22). How we think and what we think is important not only to our mental well-being but to our whole well-being—mental, physical, social and emotional. For this reason Scripture gives fundamental emphasis to the written word and, significantly, in a book on health and healing we begin, not with dance, nor with the physical, emotional or social, but with the mental aspect of our being.

When the Bible uses the term 'mind', it refers to the whole thinking man, not just the intellect. It includes the understanding and will, and often overlaps with the 'heart' which in New Testament thinking is the seat of the will, intellect and feeling. Paul wrote 'Do not conform any longer to the pattern of this world, but be transformed by the renewing of your mind. Then you will be able to test and approve what God's will is—his good, pleasing and perfect will' (Rom

12:2). 'Set your minds on things above, not on earthly things' (Col 3:2). Both represent important prerequisites for mental health and healing. The prophet no doubt had this in mind when he wrote: 'Thou wilt keep him in perfect peace, whose mind is stayed on thee' (Is 26:3, AV). Clearly, it is essential to mental health that we learn constructive thought patterns. In response to the question of the Psalmist, 'How can a young man keep his way pure?' is the reply, 'By living according to your word' (Ps 119:9).

'It is written...' is a phrase that occurs many times throughout Scripture, and significantly so. 'Faith comes from hearing the message, and the message is heard through the word of Christ' (Rom 10:17). 'All Scripture is God-breathed and is useful for teaching, rebuking, correcting and training in righteousness' (2 Tim 3:16–17)—for *maintaining* health, *restoring* health and *preventing* dis-ease. The Psalmist said: 'The words of the Lord are flawless, like silver refined in a furnace of clay, purified seven times' (Ps 12:6), and 'Your word is a lamp to my feet and a light for my path' (Ps 119:105)—it is designed to prevent us from stumbling and falling, from being dis-eased' (see also 1 Peter 2:8). 'Great peace have they who love your law, and nothing can make them stumble' (Ps 119:165).

Traditionally, it is not unusual to consider sickness and dis-ease as something given to an afflicted person from essentially 'outside' and healing as something to be administered by another person, again from 'outside'. But contemporary medicine is increasingly coming to accept the age-old teaching of Scripture that healing, as with dis-ease, is as much if not more to do with our inner nature, and especially our minds. And the key to mental well-being lies in a faithful obedience to 'what is written'.

The mind is significantly one of Satan's greatest battle grounds and one of the major causes of much sickness and dis-ease. In my experience as a Christian involved in the performing arts, the imagination—that particularly creative part of our mental faculty—is perhaps most especially susceptible to such attacks and, ironically, what is in essence the most original and creative aspect of our mental faculty is also, potentially, the most destructive. Time and time again in my ministry of Christian dance, I have seen imagination and artistic sensitivity, essential to artistic endeavour, become the channels through which Satan has got to us to undermine ourselves and our work. Imagination at its best and most positive is excitingly productive and fulfilling, contributing wonderfully to mental, as well as general, well-being. But when it is not founded upon the written word, it can cause much harm.

> Imagination is to the emotions what illustrations are to a text; what music is to a ballad. It is the ability to form mental pictures, to visualise irritating and fearful situations in concrete form. As soon as we perceive a feeling and begin to think about it, the imagination goes to work. The imagination reinforces thoughts, the thoughts intensify the feelings and the whole business builds up. There is only one way to beat this game and that is to stop the thoughts in their tracks and blot them out of the imaginary pictures.[1]

Medical evidence would suggest that something like a third of patients in our hospitals and two thirds or more having to visit their doctors, are there because of a destructive use of imagination.

But imagination is also one of God's greatest gifts to us, as is reflected in the whole artistic tradition, and it is clear that it can contribute as much to health and healing as it can to dis-ease.

> Throughout the ages and in numerous cultures, imagination has been regarded as a powerful agent in the healing process. Unfortunately, this notion had fallen into disfavour during the

last three hundred years among western psychologists and physicians. In the seventeenth century Descartes had proposed the mind/body dualism, that the mind exists independently of the body and exerts no influence upon it. Descartes' ideas were suited to the times and he found a large and faithful following. Then, of course, the behaviourists did their part to ban imagination from the domain of legitimate concerns of psychologists.

But during the last decade the climate has changed dramatically: psychologists and physicians are again proclaiming that imagination plays a vital role in both mental and physical health; and they have furnished numerous experimental and clinical investigations to support their contention. They have shown that mental images can bring about rapid and far reaching emotional, psychological and physiological changes. In fact, it now has become clear that imaginal events can have an impact which is as forceful as that of reality.[2]

Canon Jim Glennon, writing about his unique healing ministry in Sydney, urges that in sickness and dis-ease 'we must stop affirming the problem of disease and start affirming the relevant promises, in faith.'[3]

Scripture is insistent on the need to obey the voice of conscience. Failure to do this can sometimes lead to serious consequences. By rejecting conscience some people have been shipwrecked in their faith, warns Paul in 1 Timothy 1:19. 'A clear conscience is a great step toward barricading the mind against neuroticism.'[4] 'The emphasis on sin has largely disappeared from the teachings of religion . . . at the very time when psychology has discovered its importance.'[5]

If we are to enjoy good health, we must not ignore the conscience (see Psalms 32 and 38!). What a person eats is not as important as the inner bitternesses, resentments, hurts, rejections and guilts that 'eat him'. An anti-acid tablet can never reach these acids.

The human mind is like a human body. It can be wounded.
Sorrow is a wound. It cuts deeply, but is at least a 'clean' wound,
unless it is rooted in sin. It will heal unless something gets into
it — such as the poisons of self pity and bitterness.[6]

At a recent medical conference on psychosomatic medicine a
speaker shared a story about a woman who had been seriously
wounded by her son. She was urged to forgive her son and
give up her resentments and bitternesses since they were so
obviously poisoning her whole being. She replied bitterly, 'I
would rather die!' She did. Such is the destructive power of
our minds. At the same conference many stories were told of
the extraordinary healing power of the mind as a result of
thinking positively.

In understanding the relationship between the mind and
dis-ease, it is important to recognise that thought patterns
produce feelings, and feelings produce actions. Therefore,
any permanent healing must of necessity deal with the
problems of the mind. Unless the person's thinking patterns
change, his struggle with dis-ease, whatever its form, will
continue. As one doctor put it, 'You're as healthy as your
attitudes, not just your arteries.' 'If my conscience is clouded
then my sight of him is impaired, and my faith falters. A pure
conscience is one which doing its duty faithfully, is very
sensitive to the approach of evil.' 'Whatever is true, whatever
is noble, whatever is right, whatever is pure, whatever is
lovely, whatever is admirable — if anything is excellent or
praiseworthy — think about such things' (Phil 4:8). 'Put to
death, therefore, whatever belongs to your earthly nature'
(Col 3:5).

Let us, therefore, commit ourselves to the laws of the mind
and mental health as reflected in Scripture, seeing them as
primary conditions of health and well-being. 'Blessed are the
pure in heart, for they will see God' (Mt 5:8). It is as vital for
us to pray, 'Create in me a pure heart, O God, and renew a

steadfast spirit within me' (Ps 51:10) as it was for David all those many hundreds of years ago.

Dance and mental health

In what sense can it be argued that dance represents a means towards mental health and healing? There are two basic ways in which dance can contribute to mental well-being.

(1) Dance is a 'language', a non-verbal form of knowing and articulation, through which man can come to experience and express something of both his inner and outer, physical and metaphysical world.

(2) Dance as a physical activity can contribute significantly to mental well-being, as research into sport and recreational medicine shows.

But before I approach these two major justifications for dance as a means to health and healing, it is important to say something about the nature and conditions of mental health with regard to the Christian dance ministry since the effectiveness and efficiency, in part at least, of those who take part in this ministry is related to their own mental well-being. We need, too, to look at the nature and conditions of mental health with regard to the church.

The nature and conditions of mental health as it relates to the dance ministry

First of all we have to acknowledge the fundamental importance of founding such a ministry on the written word of Scripture. The key to mental health lies in the written word, and everything that has so far been said about mental health can be applied to the Christian dance group. I cannot stress this enough. Again and again, I have watched performing arts teams of all sorts stumble and fall because of ignorance or neglect of this fundamental principle. I, too, have fallen many times as a consequence of neglecting such a focus. All too often, in my experience, such ministries are built upon the sand of youthful ideas and enthusiasms, whose focus tends to be more on dance—on technique, choreography and repertoire, on the joy and excitement of intimate fellowship, 'being on the road', being a part of the church family as a whole—than upon a disciplined and mature commitment to the written word. I do not want to undermine or underestimate the importance of these other motives or deny the extraordinary effectiveness of ministries that come from such energetic enthusiastic and committed teams. I simply want to emphasise the proper, healthy and lasting base for such a ministry. The Christian dance group must be rooted first of all in a faithful commitment and obedience to the written word, worked out and lived daily in the life of such a ministry. *How* we live our life, *how* we work out our faith together, within the fellowship, is—in the end—the true nature of the ministry. And if the dance ministry is to be concerned with health and healing, then it is of fundamental importance that the team is basically healthy (see Matt 5:23).

Another important foundation of a dance ministry, and one that young people sometimes find very difficult to understand, is a disciplined scriptural acknowledgement of our own fallenness, our own state of dis-ease and our own need of healing. All too often in youthful ministries there is an admirable concern for truth but little regard for compassion. Compassion, the essence of Jesus' ministry, must be a central core of any healing ministry. And compassion, it seems to me, can only come from the profound painful experience of personal dis-ease. Our acknowledgement of our own basically sinful nature has to be experienced and worked out within the fellowship of such a ministry day by day. There will be, there must be, many failures, hurts, disappointments and dis-illusionments as you seek authenticity in your life—both personally and collectively, as you come to recognise your own brokenness and sinfulness. But these failings and hurts will, eventually, become the building blocks of growth and redevelopment for the team. They should be seen, therefore, as essential and positive growth points upon which to found a strong and healthy ministry. All too frequently we shy away from such behaviours. We see them as failures. We pretend that they don't exist and try desperately to behave super-spiritually, until we explode. We become disillusioned, deeply hurt and disappointed with each other—and usually disband!

With all that you do and experience as a team you must keep your eyes focused upon him through the written word, obeying in faith—irrespective of your own 'deceitful heart's logic'—the laws of health and healing. The word of the Lord will be your rock. I speak as one who has had to learn this painfully and as one who is still learning it—painfully! In the end, the Christian faith is not about dance, about enthusiasms of the heart, about good feelings, good deeds and successful performances . . . as important as all those are. No, in the end—and at the beginning—the Christian faith is an obedience, *in faith*, to the written word. There are going to be times when you will be down—physically, emotionally, mentally and socially. These are the times especially when you will be unable to rely on your own thinking and feeling. At such times of tiredness and irritability, the 'devil prowls around like a roaring lion looking for someone to devour', and it is only a faithful obedience to the written word that will save the ministry from dis-ease and destruction. And when, in fact, you do fail to obey—and alas you will—it will be the written word especially that will restore you and the team to health and healing. Feelings and moods of the heart, body and fellowship—especially the Christian dance fellowship with all the sensitivities and vulnerabilities that are part of being an artist, a dancer and a Christian 'on the road'—are fallible and unreliable. They will let you down; they are sand. Your rock is the written word.

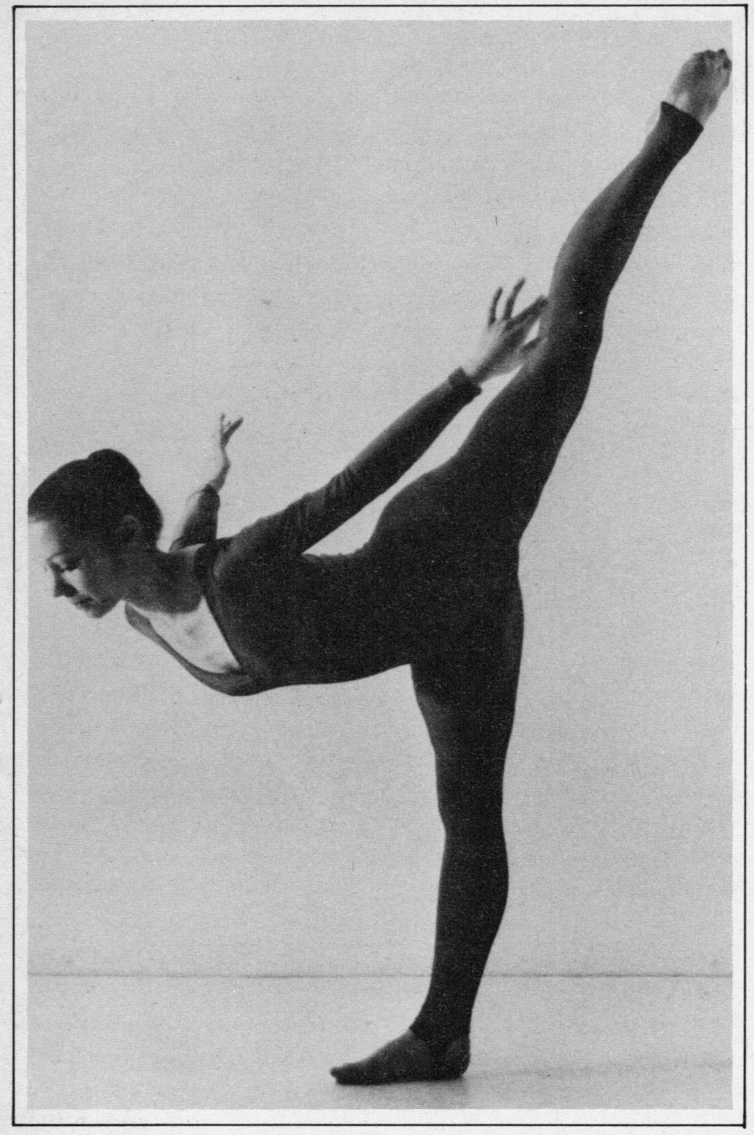

'*Honour God with your body*' (1 Cor 6:20).

The nature and conditions of mental health with regard to dance and the church

Reluctantly it has to be admitted that within the church as a whole there exists some considerable mental dis-ease with regard to dance and the Christian faith. For many it still represents a stumbling block. The problem, I feel, is not so much Scripture as education. All too often congregations simply do not understand the nature and conditions of dance and all too often, as dancers, we fail to communicate because we fail to educate. This is precisely what Christian Dance Ministries (CDM) was especially set up to do: to educate, describe and explain within a disciplined context of Scripture, and to encourage a dialogue within the church as to the nature and conditions of dance.

If dance is to be restored to its rightful and lawful place within the church one of the first concerns of dance must be to make meaningful, what for many is a foreign language. As Paul says, 'Unless you speak intelligible words with your tongue, how will anyone know what you are saying? You will just be speaking into the air. Undoubtedly there are all sorts of languages in the world, yet none of them is without meaning. If then I do not grasp the meaning of what someone is saying, I am a foreigner to the speaker, and he is a foreigner to me' (1 Cor 14:9–11).

To return, then, to our justification of dance as a means towards mental health and healing: dance is a 'language', a non-verbal form of knowing and articulation, through which man can come to experience and express his being.

In a world dominated by words, by propositional knowledge and discursive truths, we can easily be misled into thinking that verbal language systems are the only way of expressing and experiencing truth. But this is nonsense, logically and empirically! It is an everyday fact, as Scripture says, that 'Undoubtedly there are all sorts of languages in the world, yet none of them is without meaning.' No one 'language', no one system of expression and communication, has the exclusive right to the truth or the monopoly over truth. All systems of thought and feeling have a rightful place within a total knowledge of the faith. Dance, along with all the other non-verbal expressive arts such as music, painting, sculpture, architecture and design has a legitimate place within man's thinking.[7] Although undoubtedly the written and spoken word is a fundamental and essential form of public communication—and nowhere more so than in Scripture—it is but one of many languages through which man can come to experience and express himself.

With regard to the faith, I am reminded that 'The word is never as mighty as the thought which makes it. We realise this as we reject certain words as unsuitable to the thought we had in generating them.' 'God is not unknowable by the mind, but He is unutterable, which is not the same thing,' remarks Rene Williams.[8]

Too often our notion of faith is falsified by our emphasis on the statements *about* God which faith believes. The statements, the propositions, which faith accepts on the divine authority are media through which one passes in order to reach the divine truth. It is, of course, true that theology can and must study the intellectual content of revealed truth. But this is not the final object of faith. Phoenix reminds us that languages are potentially bridges or barriers to knowing and understanding, depending upon the sort of things one seeks to know. They are rather like the paradigms referred to earlier in our discussion of contemporary medicine. The language of science, for example, may constitute an invaluable bridge to coming to know and understand the anatomy and physiology of our body, but a barrier when it comes to knowing and understanding our spiritual being.

Understanding language means, in part, coming to understand the limitations as well as the strengths, the appropriateness and inappropriateness of various symbolic systems.

This, to my mind, is an important aspect of mental health. Coming to acknowledge and understand the limitations of our human languge systems is rather like recognising our brokenness before God, because we are informed by educational physchologists that we use something like less than 10% of our brain potential! What will we know when we realise to the full our mental potential? Jung once wrote, 'The world beyond is a reality, an *experiential fact*. We only don't understand it.' This lack of understanding is in part, I believe, a reflection of the limitations of human languages.

> Sometimes we are so obsessed with verbal correctness that we never go beyond words to the ineffable reality which they attempt to convey. The living God, The God who is God, and not a philosopher's abstraction, lies infinitely beyond the reach of anything our eyes can see or our minds can understand."[9]

The language of dance, like the language of music, deals above all with the ineffable, that which is not describable in terms of words. It is, moreover, essentially 'presentational' rather than '*re*-presentational'. It deals not so much with what is, but with what is to be.[10] Today, as always, the unique secret forces of the arts can help reveal and awaken much of what is unexpressed and unknown, dormant in man. Aaron Copeland, the contemporary American composer, writing about the spiritual nature that is in every man, says: 'A masterwork awakens in us reactions of a spiritual order that are already in us, only awaiting to be aroused.' Music and dance are means of God's grace through which we can grow in awareness of that spiritual nature which is in us. This is very much the thinking behind the music of Taizé — that extraordinary ecumenical community in France, with its unique expression of spirituality in music. While rooted in Scripture, the music at Taizé is created to express a spirituality that words themselves cannot and are not meant to do. It evokes an atmosphere appropriate to the spiritual dimensions of understanding and experiencing.

This is the position that the English music mystic Ralph Vaughan-Williams takes up when he says of music: 'The object of all art is to obtain a partial revelation of that which is beyond human senses and human faculties—of that which is spiritual.' The human, visible, audible and intellectual media which artists of all kinds use, are symbols not of other visible and audible things (ie 'representational'—see Langer), but of what lies beyond sense and knowledge (ie 'presentational').

Bruno Walter wrote: 'I do not believe that man is given any more immediate access to the feeling of the logos and its activities than through music which is the resounding message of its divine creative, all organising being.'

'Through art humanity creates forms in which the spirit finds expression. Forms made by man in architecture, sculpture, painting, music and poetry are all scope for the spirit to reveal itself.'[11]

And what of dance? In what way does dance express spiritual truth? Let us look at what some of the early Modern Dance pioneers themselves have said.

Doris Humphrey writes:

> People on the whole are slaves of 'the word' and the tendency is to believe that if it cannot be written it cannot be said at all . . . the exclusive expression of the Self through the medium of words, which certainly are indispensable for the ordering of groceries, or the writing of a treatise on political economy, but in my opinion are by no means able to express the whole of man. The dancer believes his art has something to say which cannot be expressed in words or in any other way than dancing. There are times when the simple dignity of movement can fulfil the function of a volume of words. There are movements which impinge upon the nerves with a strength that is incomparable for movement has power to stir the sense and emotions unique to itself.

Ted Shawn, a professional dancer who originally trained for the priesthood and was, with Ruth St Dennis, intimately concerned with sacred dance, writes,

> Religion is a matter of feeling not intellect, and every spiritual teacher has complained at some time or another of the limitations of the language of written or spoken word. It is not a question of *saying* but *being* and the finest expression of Being is through the dance.

Mary Wigman observes:

> The dance is a living language which speaks of man — an artistic message soaring above the ground of reality in order to speak, on a higher level, in images and allegories of man's innermost emotions and need for communion. It might very well be that, above all, the dance asks for direct communication without any detours. Because its bearer and intermediary is man himself and because his instrument of expression is the human body, whose natural movement forms the material for the dance, the only material which is his and his own to use.

Martha Graham writes:

> Man expressed his noblest self in dance and gesture, until the word-mongers put him to sleep with their dreary drugs and grabbed the ordering and governance of ritual for themselves. The word was made more important than the act so that now religion is a doleful mumbling in church pews and the philosophy of life is a tangle of incomprehensible phrases in a book. The dancer and artist deplores the tendency to restrict the expression of the grandest impulses of humanity to agitations in the larynx and to words.

Virginia Stewart writes:

> The modern dance is an expression through an irrational medium

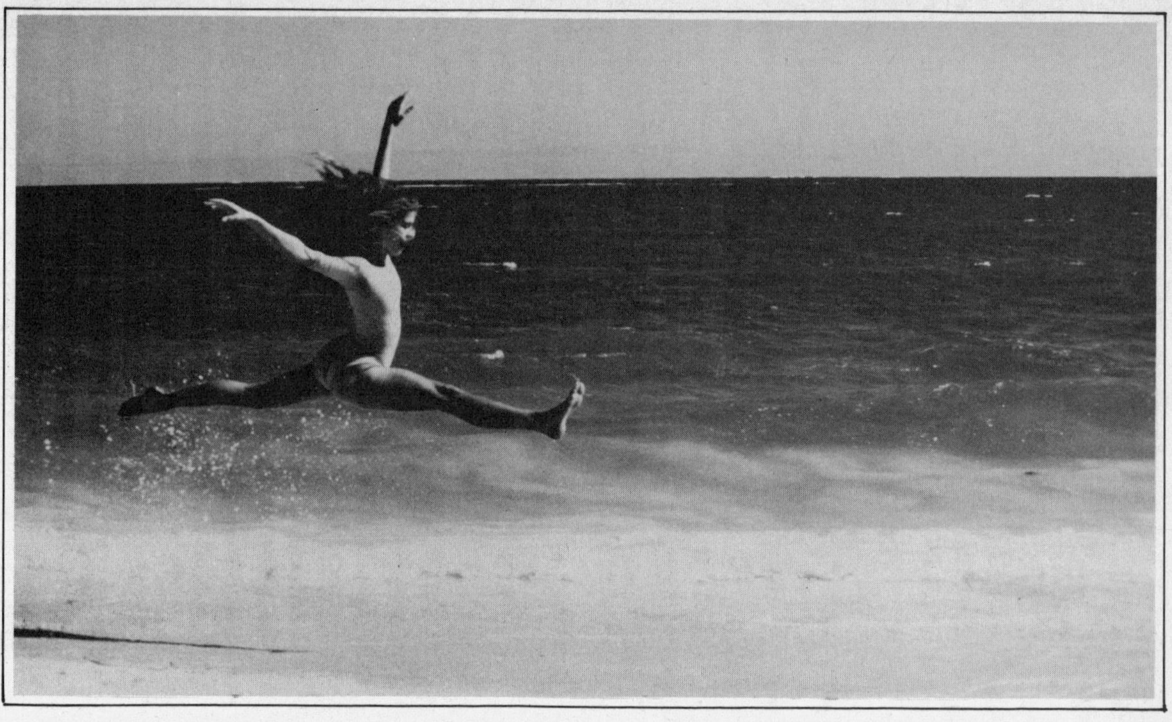

'My heart leaps for joy and I will give thanks to him in song (Ps 28:4). Rejoice and be glad' (Mt 5:12).

of bodily movement of the grasped but inarticulate emotional and intellectual experiences which man, in the whole history of his culture, has never been able to convert into words. If the spiritual content, the meaning of dance, could be converted into words it could be better written than danced. It is the high purpose of the dance to convert these intangible mental urges, these deeply felt but inexplicable emotions into movement.

Glen Tetley says:

> One of the hardest things to do is to put dance into words, because it exists on a level that is pre-word. (Pre-sentational as opposed to re-presentational).

John Cranko, in answering the question, 'What does it mean to create dances?' replied 'I think it means total expression of the things that one cannot say with words...one's whole life, what one is, one's being, without being able to define them. I suppose if one could define them, one would be a writer. To try and find that thing which movement says, is what no other art can find.'

It is this inability to translate the meaning of dance creations into words, and the very fact that the feelings aroused by these creations in the spectators are seldom identical, that gives the modern dance its greatest and strongest raison d'etre. Movement, the substance of dance, reveals that inexpressible residue of emotion which cannot be conveyed through words.

In the spirit of the Quaker spirituality, 'may our hearts and bodies be our ears'.[12]

One of the most important writers and articulators of dance is Susan Langer who argues that, 'The primary function of art [dance] is to objectify feelings so we can contemplate them and understand them. It is the formulation of our so-called inner experience, the 'inner life' that is impossible to achieve by discursive thought alone. What discursive symbolism—language in the literal sense—does for our awareness of things about us and our own relation to them, the arts do for our awareness of the subjective.'

As we have seen, imagination has an important role to play in mental health. When through the vehicle of dance the diseased approaches the cross armed with the knowledge and understanding of health and healing as revealed by Scripture; when he or she comes, claiming in faith those promises, there emerges a powerful potential for healing. Remember, steps by themselves do not constitute the dance experience. The dancer, in this case the diseased, has to invest consciously in an informed and imaginative way something of herself and her disease in those steps in order for there to be expression and communication. When this imaginative use of the mind, rooted in the word, accompanied by the faithful promises of Scripture and surrounded by the Holy Spirit is applied to the dance we begin to experience how this 'primitive' (primary) language channel of God's extraordinary power:

> When we understand the impact that faith can have on our emotions and bodies, we realise that an experience of God plays a creative role in both physical and psychological healing. Real prayer, which gives us an experience of the purpose and meaning in the universe, as well as a real knowledge of a relationship with God, can have incredible observable healing powers.[13]

Dance thus represents an invaluable contribution to mental health and well-being in that it is an avenue of consciousness, a non-verbal form of experience and expression—physical and metaphysical. It can deal, above all, with our inner being and with those things that cannot and should not be put into words.

Dance as a physical activity and mental health

Though we know that the mind can work on the body to bring about dis-ease, we sometimes forget that the body can also work on the mind. All our thoughts and feelings are inextricably interwoven with physical movement. This is the basis of dance healing. Accumulating evidence suggests that body movements not only reflect thought processes but actually help create them. Significantly in terms of dance as health and healing, neurophysiologist-biologist, Ernst Gellhan, states that emotions and thoughts can be controlled through the somatic system — that is, by willed action of the musculature. For example, there is a close association between physical tension and mental tension. When we are worried we feel tense in our body: when we relax our body very completely we soon begin to feel relaxed in our mind. Our bad temper is often a result of sheer physical tiredness. It is a well recorded fact that low physical condition can cause all sorts of mental disturbances. In the sense that dance is a physical activity it can contribute significantly to mental health and well-being.

A considerable body of research indicates a positive correlation between physical activity and mental well-being. A number of investigations have shown that regular physical activity can have a remarkable effect on overall mental health and well-being, on change in mental states and intellectual functioning. Experiments have reported a variety of mental benefits gained from regular physical activity including an increased vitality and mental energy, reduced mental tension, lower anxiety level, less nervousness, few sleep problems, less fatigue, a greater emotional stability.

One piece of research suggested that 'running in some cases can function better than psychotherapy in the treatment of moderate depression'.

Another investigation concluded that those with un-favourable mental health scores prior to physical training made a greater progress with respect to the goal of mental health, than others.

Others have reported an increase in overall well-being.

Although most of the research is related to general physical activity I believe we can legitimately apply these findings to dance in that it *is* a physical activity.

When the psyche becomes fragmented, exhausted, and dis-eased we can sometimes turn to the body as a source of healing and freeing dis-ease.

Body therapies are based on the idea that producing changes in the body on a neuromuscular level will produce not only physical but mental and emotional changes. Most of them derive from the theories of William Reich, who contended that life experiences are locked into the muscles and the skeleton structure. Most body therapies involve physical restructuring as an aid to mental and emotional processes.

Notes

1. V Callin, *Me, Myself and You* (Dodd and Mead).
2. A A Sheik Ed, *Imagination and Healing* (Baywood, 1984).
3. Jim Glennon, *How Can I Find Healing?* (Hodder and Stoughton: London, 1984).
4. W Sadler, *Practice of Psychiatry* (Simon and Schuster, 195).
5. H C Link, *None of these Diseases* (Lakeland: Basingstoke).
6. C L Allen, *God's Psychiatry* (Power Books: Old Tappan, NJ).
7. See Martin Blogg, *Dance and the Christian Faith* (Hodder and Stoughton: London, 1985).
8. A Padovan, *Contemplation and Compassion* (Peter Pauper Press, 1984).
9. Thomas Merton, *New Seeds of Contemplation* (New Directions, 1961).
10. Susan Langer, *Feeling and Form* (Routledge and Kegan Paul: London).
11. Baron A Rosenkrantz, *The Mission of Art*.
12. J M Brown Ed., *Visions of Modern Dance* (Dance Books: London.)
13. Morton Kelsey, *Healing and Christianity* (Harper and Row: London).

4

The Physical Dimension of Human Being

Scripture and physical health

Scripture is surprisingly explicit about the nature and conditions of physical health and has a great deal to say about our body.

As we have already seen (see chapter 1) our body, our physical being, is God's creation. This caused the Psalmist to write: 'I praise you because I am fearfully and wonderfully made' (Ps 139:14).

> In physical terms, nothing in the world is quite so fearfully and wonderfully made as the body. It is one of the most delicate and amazing instruments that can be imagined. It is more precise than the most perfect of man's precision instruments.[1]

David expresses a spiritual and sacred awesomeness with regard to the body, and rightly so. The body is made to express God, and perform his will. The parts of the body are to be instruments of righteousness unto God. Paul tells us 'Do you not know that your body is a temple of the Holy Spirit, who is in you, whom you have received from God? You are not your own; you were bought at a price. Therefore honour God with your body (1 Cor 6:19, 20). It is, then, with an indescribable consciousness of holiness, of fear and awe, of joy and wonder that the believer can offer his body—as a *living* sacrifice of praise and thanksgiving.

As a result of the fall, our human bodies, along with all creation, became dis-eased, but they have been redeemed by the death of Jesus, and we are told to offer our bodies back to God: 'Therefore, I urge you, brothers, in view of God's mercy, to offer your bodies as living sacrifices, holy and pleasing to God—this is your spiritual act of worship. Do not conform any longer to the pattern of this world but be transformed by the renewing of your mind' (Rom 12:1). Now, with Paul, we can pray that 'now as always Christ will be exalted in my body' (Phil 1:20).

God created us by his power and redeemed us by his love. In view of his mercy surely the only fitting response is to accept ourselves, in all our humanity, acknowledging him as our originator and source, and then offer to him all our humanity?

Physical abuse and dis-ease

In focusing on the physical dimension of human being, I am anxious not to limit our thinking to physical fitness alone, the traditional concern of physical well-being, but also to consider body feeling, body expression, bodily contact, body image, touch, sensuality and sexuality. It will soon become clear that it is sometimes difficult to distinguish between these various dimensions of our physical being, especially when it comes to dance, since dance is so obviously much more than a mere physical activity. This, indeed, is one of its characteristic strengths.

Incredible as it may seem a platonic dualism still pervades much of the thinking of many Christians. They are seriously dis-eased and negatively affected by abuses of worldly think-ing, and by the sometimes rigid and fearful misplaced puri-tanical attitudes of the past. 'There are many of God's people who conscientiously walk with Him, both in spirit and soul, but seem to have a deeper inner reluctance to allow Christ control of their bodily behaviour. They act as if this were a realm outside and apart from His area of interest and influence.'[2]

Within the context of the physical dimension of our human be-ing there is some considerable need for healing. Much of the dis-ease related to the body is, in my experience, essentially the product of ignorance and lack of education. One of the keys to the restoration of physical well-being lies in education, an education rooted in Scripture and worked out in real, practical terms of the body, feelings and relationships. The body, and all that is associated with it, is God's gift to us as our earthly house as well as his temple for the few years on this earth. Let us acknowledge it as such and treat it with a gentle respect and gracious goodwill (1 Cor 6:12–20).

Physical stimulation is vital to healthy physical being, and to well-being generally. We are well aware of the serious negative effects of physical deprivation in the early years of human development. What we are not so aware of is the negative effects of physical deprivation in adult life. As children we are encouraged to move and we delight in our movement. We are also encouraged to take delight in body contact, in touching, holding, cuddling and embracing. But, somehow, as we grow older these physical experiences become less and less frequent, until many reach a point where there is no deliberate physical stimulation at all. As we will go on to see, such physical deprivation can have a serious negative effect of the whole of our being. Conversely, it will be shown that physical stimulation represents a powerful healing and therapeutic tool.

It is difficult within our society to talk about the body and dance without talking about sex. For many, sex is inseparable from the body, especially dance. I do not believe that dance is necessarily a deliberate and explicit expression of sexuality, but I do recognise that since it involves the bodies of men and women in action and in contact, it may manifest something of man's sensuous and erotic nature. While I acknowledge that for some this represents a problem, I cannot in all honesty, given what Scripture says about the body and the physical aspect of our being, see it as something inherently wrong, unlawful or evil. To see it in these terms is to see it, I believe, in misguided and dis-eased terms. 'We should recognise the principle that certain pleasures and feelings are willed us by God. We cannot live in truth if we automatically suspect all feelings and desires. It is humility, I would suggest, to accept our God given humanity, and quite proud, if not arrogant, to reject it.'[3] As C S Lewis shrewdly observes: 'All my life a ludicrous and portentous solemnisation of [the body and] sex has been going on . . . when natural things look most divine, the demoniac is just round the corner.'[4]

It can hardly be said that sex, sensuality and eroticism are irreligious. Genesis certainly makes it clear that they are part of God's purpose in the first place.

> Modesty is a beautiful thing, but the atittude which regards all that is related to the body as murky, furtive and secret is stupid, unhealthy and dangerous. If, because we have been ignorant or mistaught about our physical being, we pretend we never have feelings or desires, we banish the poor relation — physical emotion — into the unconscious: that is to say, we repress it. But the poor relation (like all suppressed feelings and emotions) does not cease to exist! He plagues us with a particularly unpleasant kind of blackmail and neurosis, and sexual perversion is sometimes the result. There is nothing evil in having physical feelings and desires. Everyone has them![5]

'The worship of the Church must first of all be natural, then it can be supernatural otherwise it could end up blatantly unnatural,' says Howard Marshall.[6] 'Pleasure,' as C S Lewis points out, 'is God's invention and not the devil's.' In spite of sin and the fall, the world remains God's good creation and it keeps its essential goodness, in which its Creator rejoiced, whatever man, in his freedom, does with it. Our first step as Christians is to thank our loving Creator that we *can* appreciate through our minds, bodies, hearts and each other, something of the beauty that *is* the body, that we can delight in the physical sensations that come from dancing.

Thomas Merton writes:

The body is neither evil nor unreal. It has a reality that is given by God and this reality is therefore holy. Hence we say rightly . . . that the body is the 'temple of God', meaning that His perfect reality is enshrined there in the mystery of our being. Let no one, then, dare to hate or despise the body that has been entrusted to him by God, and let no one dare misuse this body. Let him not desecrate his own natural unity by dividing himself, soul against body. Soul and body together subsist in the reality of the hidden, inner person. If the two are separated from one another, there is no longer a person, there is no longer a living subsisting reality made in the image and likeness of God. The 'marriage' of body and soul in one person is one of the things that makes man the image of God; and what God has joined no man can separate without danger to his sanity![7]

Many of the twentieth-century pioneers of modern dance were aware of the sacredness of the body which they regarded as a spiritual vehicle, to be treated with wonder and awe, as well as being something beautiful and sensual. Remember that the early pioneers were concerned with acknowledging and expressing the truth in man, man in all his humanity, in real life.

Physical and body dis-ease, so common among Christians, is not uncommon among professionally trained dancers, strange as it may seem. There appears to be something of a paradox here since one would have thought that the extra-ordinary intimacy and familiarity with the body which comes from working with it so hard over many years would bring a healthy ease, free of inhibition. But this is not always so. I have met and worked with dancers who have at times displayed an extraordinary dis-ease and inhibition and even fear — in personal terms — with regard to their bodies. There is often a need for sensitive healing and certainly any Christian dancer who is ill at ease with his or her body needs to acknowledge this fact and deal with it before embarking upon a ministry of dance and healing.

Body dis-ease is the product of a number of factors. It is, in part, the result of the body image that one has of oneself, and for the dancer this very often means striving and struggling for a particular image or ideal. In the process of struggling with one's body the body is seen as something separate from one's self, first because it is regarded as an ideal outside of one's true self, and secondly because one constantly feels one is pushing and punishing 'it' rather than one's self. It is as if 'the body' will not do what *we* want it to do — that it is independent of us and often, seemingly, against us. In fact, we often come to despise the body for some of these reasons. When we are unable to fulfil the ideal we hold, we consciously or unconsciously reject our bodies. Paradoxically, when we do achieve the ideal, different problems arise as a result of sometimes confusing this ideal with the real. This is perhaps particularly so with young and immature dancers. Furthermore, not only can the nature of the physical training seriously retard the physical and emotional nature of the dancer, but the usually extremely narrow and focused, rather cloistered and unworldly existence, of the dancer can often contribute to a false sense of reality, for example, the dancer has an unnatural romantic image of himself. This frequently leads to social and emotional disease.

We know, from our knowledge of holistic medicine, that anything we do to one aspect of our human being affects all the others. When we as dancers punish and abuse our physical bodies this is inevitably reflected in our minds and our hearts, as well as in our relationships with other people. In describing something of this extraordinary abuse by the dancer, Annabel Ferriman says: 'It is sad that these people whom we worship as the acme of physical beauty are being subjected to so much [dis-ease] and disorder. In most cases there is a contradiction between living a complete healthy life and being a dancer!'

Body dis-ease, as we have seen, is also the consequence of living in an ungodly world, and there is no more ungodly world than that of the theatre. I have known professionally trained dancers come into the Christian world feeling very confused and dis-eased as a result of fears and inhibitions arising from both training and experiences that go to make up the secular world of entertainment. To those who are experiencing something of this dis-ease, let me urge you to look at what Scripture says about you and your body, and by implication, dance. Let me also assure you that the abuse of a good thing—dance and the body—is not sufficient reason for its non-use. Quite the opposite, it is every reason for the Christian to restore both to their rightful use.

St Dennis writes:

> In modern times we have used almost exclusively the language of the intellect—speech—to express all states and stages of our consciousness, and by so doing we have inhibited and dwarfed the physical and emotional beauty of the self, not knowing that dancing in its nobler uses is the very temple and word of the living spirit. It is largely from error that the sense of separation between body and spirit has grown. Spiritual consciousness has sought entirely other means for its expression.

Martha Graham writes:

> To express what is the most moral, healthful and beautiful in art—that is the mission of the dancer. The dancer of the future

will be one whose body and soul have grown so harmoniously together that the natural language of that soul will have become the movement of the body. The dancer will not belong to a nation but to all humanity. She will dance not in the form of nymph, nor fairy, nor coquette, but in the form of a woman in her greatest and purest expression. She will realise the mission of woman's body and the holiness of all its parts.

Louis Fuller writes:

In the dance, and there ought to be a word better adapted to the thing, the human body should, despite conventional limitations, express all the sensations or emotions that it experiences. The human body is ready to express, and it would express if it were at liberty to do so, all sensations just as the body of an animal.

Limon writes:

The dancer is most fortunate indeed, for he has for his instrument the most eloquent and miraculous of all instruments the human body. . . . We explore the possibilities and potentialities inherent in every part of the body. These are the rich resources of the body. These are the voices. They must be disciplined and developed so that they can speak with truth and power . . . this highly trained responsible instrument we dedicate to a single idea: that the dance is a serious, adult art, every bit as serious as music, painting, literature and poetry.

Eric Hawkins writes:

Ever since I was a little boy living in my own culture I couldn't help but sense that something was not quite right; that all the answers had not yet been given, that something had not yet been born that desperately needed to be born. It was too much a culture of deadness and deathliness and ugly bodies. I have always wondered whether every child as he or she grows up arrives at a strange and sorrowful disillusionment when he sees the miracle of the body spoiled and degraded in the adult world. Our only image really for the body is equated with pornography. Our image of dance has always been of something we could never be — that of the fat sultan owning his pretty little dancing girls.

Hanya Holm writes:

> What you are capable of is so marvellous that it is almost impossible to imagine what you could do if you achieved it. Don't say you can never get there. Get as far as you can with a full heart and with full conviction, then try to drive on a little further. To achieve something takes strength. You are not born with strength, you have to gain it. Don't look at your exercises as something to make your muscles hurt, but as something that will make you improve yourself. Know that you are a human being, that you are able to take life as it is. Life is not an escape. It is not an excuse. It is not idle cowardice.

Mary Wigman writes:

> The ultimate and noblest meaning of the dance can have one aim only: the living work of art presented through the human body as its instrument of expression.[8]

It is clear from our discussion that the body of the Christian is a sacred trust to be surrendered and sanctified by the Lord: 'The body is . . . for the Lord, and the Lord for the body' (1 Cor 6:13). If the body is for the Lord, and dance is for the Lord, then it matters what we do with it. Do we, as Christians and as dancers, take seriously the biblical affirmation that our bodies are temples of the Holy Spirit? Do we really care for our body in such a way that it glorifies and honours God? Is it a fitting place for the Lord to dwell?

When in quiet and serious meditation we come to recognise the awesomeness of some of these scriptural principles and apply them in practical everyday life, our attitudes become radically altered. As Christians we need to pay attention to our bodies, and not just for the sake of the body alone, but because what we do or do not do to our bodies will affect our minds, spirits, emotions and social relationships as well.

Dance and physical health

Physical exercise and fitness

Whatever dance is, or is not, it is an activity which includes the body. I say 'include' because, as we have consistently emphasised, dance involves the whole being. But dance is, first of all, a physical activity and in that sense it can contribute significantly to physical fitness. Just as the condition of the mind can greatly affect the body, so, too, can the condition of the body greatly affect the mind. Both are intimately related.

In terms of physical fitness, it is essential that we do with our bodies what God intended us to do with them. One of the most fundamental, natural and God-given laws is that the functional efficiency of an organ or system improves with use and regresses with disuse, *Use it or lose it* is a biological law, the application of which has, traditionally at least, received very little attention where the human body is concerned. For example, when a joint is not used over a period of time it begins to 'freeze' or lock. Surrounding muscle will simultaneously atrophy, thus increasing the immobility, which in turn can lead to further difficulties like demineralising of the bones. In contrast, regular physical activity can lead to an increase in mineral content and greater mechanical efficiency, strength and flexibility. One can literally die from inactivity! As a result of exercise, vital energy is increased and preserved, nerves relaxed, sleep improved, and glands and vital centres toned up. When the body is in good working order, conditioned and calmed, much of the distress in the body as well as in the mind, emotions and relationships, will disappear.

Dance represents a unique physical exercise experience through which the individual, *at any age and in any condition,* can improve the functioning and general well-being of the body. In dance the mind, the emotions and others are brought into the experience. It is a truly holistic hygiene.

It is not my intention to give a detailed analysis of the nature and conditions of exercises as a contribution to well-being. For those who wish to pursue this, I have included details in the bibliography of some excellent books. Research is overwhelmingly in support of physical exercise as a necessary requisite of health. It can be argued that dance, as a regular and intelligently organised activity, leads to physical health and well-being which include the following:

Improved muscle toning, strength, precision, endurance and control
improved co-ordination, precision, balance and control of the body
improved kinaesthetic awareness
improved cardio-vascular system (heart and muscle system)
improved lung capacity and overall efficiency
improved nervous system and psyche
improved circulation
postponement of body deterioration
purification of the physical body, efficient elimination of body waste
improved weight control
improved digestive system
improved bone mineral content
improved energy, vitality and general alertness...a marked reduction of listlessness and fatigue
relaxation, calming and freeing of tension

Research into physical exercise also confirms the contribution of regular exercise towards the relieving of such diseases as:

insomnia
menstrual strain and menstrual cramps
arthritis
neuromuscular hypertension
stress-related diseases — including cancer
low back pain
weight and obesity
biochemical processes
mental and emotional disease
coronary heart disease
blood pressure and hypertension
rehabilitation

An excellent research supplement entitled *Physical Activity and Health* published in 1982 by the Scandinavian Journal of Social Medicine provides detailed evidence of the benefits of physical experience under the following headings:

(1) Consequences for health on physical INactivity

(2) Consequences for health on physical ACTivity

heart and circulation
skeleton
joints, cartilage, tendons and ligaments
nervous system
muscles and metabolism
biochemical changes in physical activity
menstrual cycle, pregnancy and birth

(3) Physical activity in treatment and rehabilitation of various patient groups.

The following extract from an article written for students, comments clearly on the health considerations of an exercise programme. It identifies at least five types of health benefits which have been attributed to exercise: strengthening the

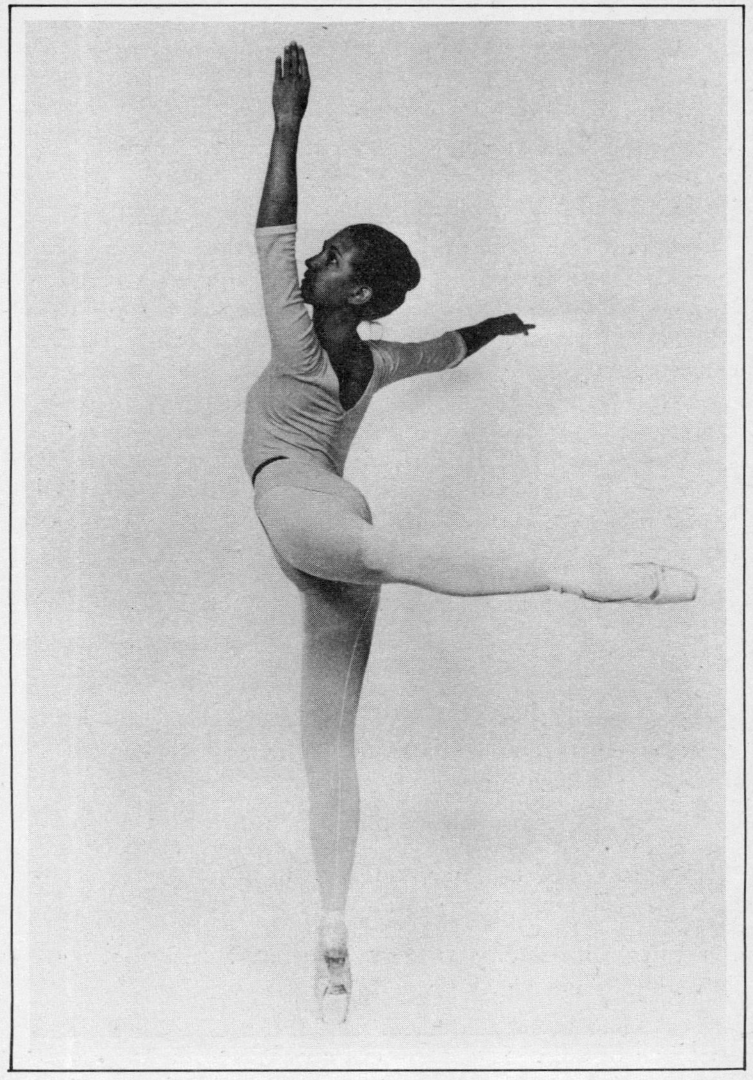

'I will give thanks unto thee, for I am fearfully and wonderfully made: marvellous are thy works, and that my soul knoweth right well' (Ps 139:13).

heart and keeping the blood vessels open; regulating meta-bolic functions, such as control of sugar; combating anxiety or depression; bolstering the immune defence, and strengthening bone and muscle.

The article goes on to say:

> What exercise really affects are factors such as blood pressure, cholesterol, blood sugar, body fat and reactions to stress; reduction in heart disease is thought to follow. Regular exercise, for example, lowers blood pressure—a major risk factor—in the majority of people, and mild hypertension can at times be treated with exercise alone. Apart from its crucial role in protecting the heart, exercise has other significant benefits, such as strengthening the muscles and skeleton to protect them from injury in later life. By increasing bone density, exercise helps prevent osteoporosis, an affliction of so many older women particularly.[9]

To summarise all that has been said in relation to physical exercise and physical well-being I will quote M Bricklin:

> If there is one supreme natural therapy for chronic and degenerative disorders, it is exercise. And if there is one natural therapy that is more natural than any other, that too is exercise.[10]

It is one of the prime tasks of physical 'health' and 'healing' to see that the organic state of the body is kept in good repair and to enhance its functional efficiency. Dance as physical exercise, if used rightly, can be used to maintain, improve, arrest, prevent and reverse a whole range of serious debilitating dis-eases.

The Scandinavian Journal of Social Medicine supplement 29, (1982) concludes on a very encouraging positive note with regard to physical activity and health:

> It has been shown that the capacity for training of the organism

is very great, and that this trainability is preserved in high degree even during illness. The consequence is that the very great majority of individuals can, through physical activity, improve their functional condition and therefore their total life situation. This holds good not only for healthy people but also for individuals with a long series of chronic illness and functional handicaps, and it also holds good at almost any age.

This conclusion is important because it reminds us that dance is not exclusively a sport activity of the young. It is for *all* people, of *all* ages. What is most encouraging is that research indicates that its benefits are significantly higher for the older age range whatever their condition, than for the younger!

I read with great interest an article by Liz Lerman, Director of 'Dancers of the Third Age'—a senior adult performing group. She writes: 'I have always felt that dance belongs to everybody. I've felt that working with seniors—with what they can contribute to and what they can gain from dance— has been seriously missing in the professional dance world.'[11]

Ruth St Dennis writes:

The spectacle of a singer or dancer or actor continuing on the stage in parts too young for him is tragic enough but still more tragic is the situation of the artist who, in his maturity, having grown to the most interesting and beautiful stage of his consciousness, is forced to withdraw from his active career because of the childish demand of the public for mere youth. Some day our consciousness will expand to take in, with the loveliness and freshness of youth, the graciousness and dignity of age, in art as well as in life. Here the dance will unfold many truths of being, many unknown or unseen joys possible to us in the very midst of our common days.

Old age, then, need not be a limiting factor in physical exercise—quite the opposite. Old people benefit physically,

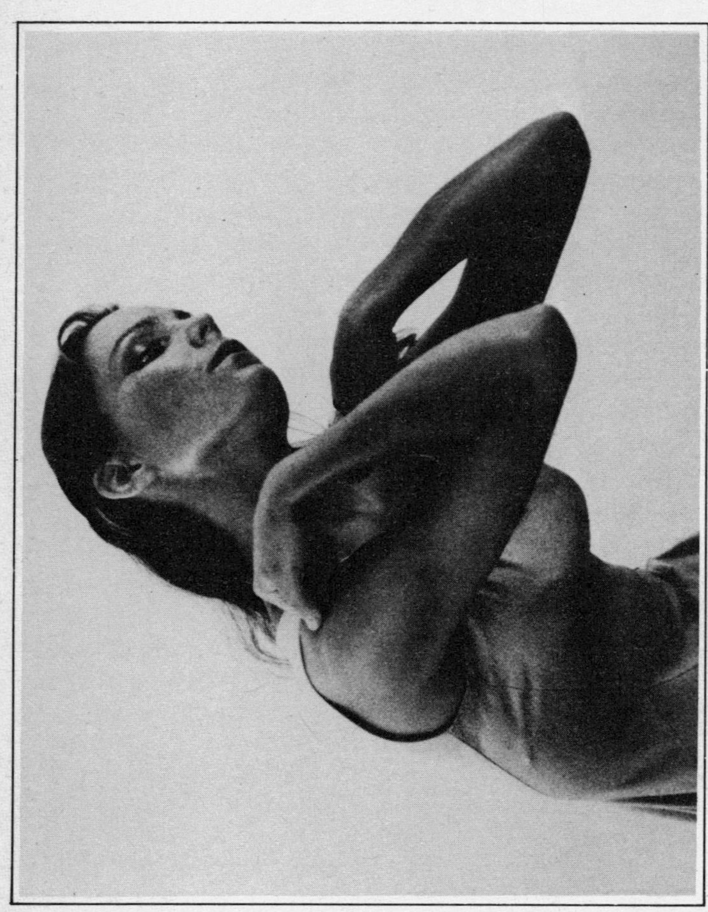

'My soul is in anguish. How long, O Lord, how long?' (Ps 6:3).

emotionally, socially and mentally from exercise.

Finally, Selwyn Hughes, in answering the question, 'Are the results of taking care of God's temple, and treating it with the respect it deserves, worth it?' gives a resounding yes. 'In addition to improved appearance, new buoyancy and greater effectiveness, you will have the gratifying sense that you have fulfilled your responsibility as the caretaker of God's temple.[12]

Physical exercise and stress

Having identified in general terms something of the beneficial nature of dance as exercise, I would now like to look in more detail into some specific dis-eases. First, I want to look at stress, one of the most common and among the most dangerous of contemporary dis-ease.

The stress that I am concerned with is not so much physical stress, as expressed in the aches and pains which arise from the misuse of the body—a not uncommon phenomenon in the dance world—but rather the stress which, while manifesting itself in the body, has its roots in a combination of deprivations arising from the predominantly sedentary nature of our life. As we have seen with regard to mental health, attitudes have physical effects. The British Medical Society states that 'not a single cell of the body is totally removed from the influence of the mind and emotions. Mind and emotion affect muscle tone. All of us no doubt have felt our muscles tighten when we become frightened, frustrated or angry. Tightened muscles can produce severe pain and dis-ease, as can be seen in chronic patients. Tension, headaches and migraine stem in part at least, from head and neck muscles in spasm. Nearly all negative emotions tend to result in physical body tension. This tension then causes pain, pain causes fatigue and fatigue results in tension, thus completing a vicious circle!'

Unrelieved tension can cause considerable harm in the individual, and sometimes even death. It can actually change the hormonal structure of the body. Muscular tension squeezes off blood circulation, creating chronic shallow breathing and reducing the amount of oxygen reaching the heart.

> Although the emotional and mental significance of muscular tension is still not fully understood, one thing that is understood and accepted is that these tensions, which grip the body, mould it, split it and distort it—must be eliminated before one can achieve inner freedom and this must be achieved before any real progress is made in verbal therapy. [13]

One way to reduce chronic unrelieved tension is to involve oneself in regular physical exercise. Through vigorous sustained movement—usually simple patterns or sequences of events that do not have too much cognitive distraction, such as walking, running, stretching, jogging, or the simple actions of aerobics—body dis-ease and malfunction can be greatly reduced and a general sense of well-being experienced.

Sometimes these tensions or blockages are the result of a deep and long process of suppression which has become habitual, so much so that it is sometimes difficult for the dis-eased to be released from it, even though he wants to be. Frequently the relieving of such armourings and blockages is an important preliminary to the healing process. Reich, one of the early pioneers in body psychology, described this situation as 'defence-armouring'. Reich theorised that personal defences were rooted in the body as chronic muscular tension. He stated that 'every increase of muscular tones in the direction of rigidity indicates that a vegetative excitation, anxiety or sexuality has become bound up.' [14] He suggested that tension in specific parts of the body relates to the attempt to resolve emotional problems by physical repression. 'Holding' in the chest area, for example, is considered indicative of repressed feelings, of needing and longing.

Most dance therapists believe that one of their major functions is to help the individual dancer reduce emotional/mental muscular tension. Through the dance experience it is possible to mobilise the chronically held areas of the dis-eased and thus begin to release through expression many repressed needs and feelings.

As E Rosen reminds us: 'There is nothing new in the idea of relieving psychic energy and tension through activity. Much of the teaching of Yoga, Zen and other Eastern systems have focused on physical and mental training as a means of achieving control of self.'[15]

> Research does prove fairly conclusively that physical exercise, whatever its form, does have a favourable effect on level of anxiety and release from tension, that it does lead to a reduction in physiological activation and a reduction in emotional reactivity and strain . . . as well as an increase in overall well-being, better sleeping habits and less depression.[16]

Physical exercise and body image

At the beginning of this chapter we spoke at some length about the physical dimension of human be-ing and the way worldly attitudes have been allowed to colour our Christian attitudes. We saw that Scripture is quite unequivocal in its view that the body is basically and originally good, created by God in his own image. It was recognised that any notion of unclean lies not in the body but in the mind and attitude of the onlooker. We have seen that Paul urges us to be transformed by the renewing of our minds and by so doing to restore the body to its rightful and lawful place.

Attitudes towards the body are frequently the same as attitudes towards dance and vice versa. Both are intimately related. Dance is a bodily expression. In restoring the body to its rightful place within Scripture we restore, by implication, the dance. In my experience it is usually easier to restore the body and the physical nature of our human being through the dance than it is through the body in itself. Within the secure and imposed structures of the dance, I have found that people are more able to expose themselves and make themselves vulnerable, physically, emotionally and socially. This is particularly so with regard to dance technique where there is not such an obvious need for a subjective and emotional involvement.

In the same way that our body affects the mind, the mind affects the body. Accordingly, once the mind begins to grasp the scriptural truth *about* the body and begins to translate those truths into firsthand practical experiences *of* the body, a much more meaningful and realistic understanding of the body emerges. The thinking or mental aspect of our knowing is balanced by a physical, emotional and, in the case of dance, social knowing. Each reinforces the other. True knowledge of Scripture will lead us into a balanced knowledge and understanding of mind, body and 'heart'—surrounded by the Holy Spirit. So, too, with regard to one's attitude towards body image.

Body image is defined as 'the impression an individual has about his or her body'. 'The person's body image is intimately related to the person's self-concept.'[17] Body image has a powerful influence on our whole being and how we experience ourselves and the outside world. How we think about the body, its shape, size and weight; how we react to other people's bodies; what we wear and how we 'display' ourselves, says an awful lot about how we perceive ourselves and our bodies and how we perceive others. Body image, then, is an important subject for the dance therapist.

In dance technique there is a deliberate and formal concern to bring about changes in body image. Both the process of exercising and the product of exercising have valuable contributions to the dis-eased. First, as already mentioned, there is a secure and formal social, emotional and physical structure within which to work, and the work is carried out with others who are concerned with the same problem. Secondly, is the well-known fact that improved functioning and appearance of the body can contribute enormously to a greater sense of self-worth, self-esteem, a greater freedom and confidence. 'As the individual gains new control and new understanding about his and others' bodies, he begins to acquire new feelings and new attitudes towards the body and towards himself.'[18]

Dance therapy, then, is concerned with creating a healthy body image—physically, emotionally and socially; with restoring the body to its rightful and lawful place in the mind and heart of the individual.

Through the dance, through exploring the body in movement, choreography and self-expression, a healthy holistic awareness of the self begins to emerge. As we become more intimately aware, more familiar, more in touch, in both physical and emotional terms, with our body, so there begins to develop a greater sense of well-being and freedom from dis-ease. Once the body has come to know the truths of Scripture in practical and experiential terms, a corresponding understanding develops in mental terms. That is the basis of dance therapy.

Physical well-being and nutrition

A discussion on nutrition right in the middle of a book on dance as health and healing may seem a little out of place. Just how can nutrition be related to dance and health? First, it should be recognised that we *are*, to a large extent, what we eat—or more significantly perhaps, in the case of the dance, what we do not eat!

It is increasingly believed that personality is a key factor with regard to health and dis-ease, but it is by no means accepted that it is wholly so. As one researcher remarked: 'People tend to go overboard and believe personality is a decisive factor in illness, when it is but one of the factors. What makes me nervous about this over-emphasis is that it makes people feel guilty when they get sick.'[19] Nutrition is basic to all aspects of our human be-ing, since it provides the building blocks and fuel for all biological processes. Every breath we take, every thought we think, every nerve impulse that triggers a beat of our heart, requires energy, and this is provided by the food we eat.

The sources of the physiological, mental, emotional and social changes in the personality are not altogether fully understood but it is clear that nutritional deficiencies, together with endocrine malfunctioning, allergic states, and drug/toxic reactions can seriously affect all these aspects of the personality.

B Strickland and K Kendall write:

Whilst clinicians are aware that medical problems or illnesses can result from behavioural and emotional difficulties, they may be less sophisticated about the reverse phenomenon. Data accumulated from a wide variety of psychiatric and psychological health delivery services do suggest that a significant proportion of clients who present themselves to mental health facilities are actually suffering from physical problems.[20]

Anxiety, irritability, memory loss, confusion, impaired concentration, depression, hearing voices, are examples of *mental* disease arising from nutritional deficiency.

Fatigue, hyper- and hypo-activity, headaches, aches and pains, bone pain, difficulty in walking, and muscle weakness are examples of *physical* disease arising from nutritional deficiency.

Nutritional deficiency is a common dis-ease among dancers, although rarely intelligently acknowledged or understood either by the dancer or teacher. Vitamin B deficiency is the one deficiency that most dancers acknowledge can lead to anxiety, irritability, loss of memory, nervousness and depression. Not an uncommon diagnosis among dancers! Vitamin D deficiency can lead to bone pain, difficulty in walking, and muscle weakness.

All these stresses and strains on top of the physical, emotional, intellectual and social stresses that go to make up the life of a dancer can be especially crippling. But it is not just vitamin deficiency that can lead to disease. Some foods and drinks have ingredients that cause disease. I am reminded of the vast quantities of soft drinks and coffee that are drunk by the dancer. We are now coming to understand, for example, that the caffeine, which is in coffee and some soft drinks, can have a powerful effect upon physiological stress response mechanisms and psychological stress. Normally caffeine is associated with symptoms of anxiety and headaches, but more recently research reveals that it is linked with depression as well. I myself know only too well the possible negative effects of caffeine in its soft drink form. While on tour of North-West Australia, cooped up in our non-air conditioned station wagon, covering vast distances in the heat and dust, working within a lonely, unfamiliar and not infrequently hostile world, we almost lived on 'cola'. It quenched our thirst and seemed to staunch our misery, irritabilities and nervousness. In hindsight it just may be that the sustained tensions, irritabilities, confusions, and depressions that characterised much of our tour could in part be attributed to large doses of caffeine. We were in fact feeding our dis-ease rather than quenching it! Interestingly enough, one major cola company has now produced a non-caffeine cola!

All these findings, and many more, remind us of the subtle intimacies and inter-relations of physical, mental, emotional and social well-being. If you as a dancer are lacking drive and energy, are irritable, tired, listless, run-down, not coping with your dancing, it could be as much to do with what you are eating or what you are not eating, as it could be with your mind, body, emotions or the group you are involved with.

Certainly, a proper diet will greatly contribute to general well-being.

For maximum physical fitness which is essential to dance, there must be adequate amounts of proteins, carbohydrates, fats, minerals, vitamins and water. If the diet is deficient in these areas there will be a marked deterioration in the ability to perform physical tasks. The vitamin B complex has been especially studied in relation to physical effort, and it is clear that a vitamin B deficiency has a particularly significant effect on physical ability—as most dancers and sportsmen know only too well. Most dancers need to boost their intake of vitamin B.

Still thinking of the dancer, some interesting studies have been done on the importance of breakfast and physical health. W W Turtle and others of the College of Medicine of the State University of Iowa have identified the important negative effects of ignoring breakfast or eating an inferior one. They noted that it resulted in a significant decrease in ability to perform physical work.[21] It has long been established that a low sugar content in the blood, which is normal following sleep, can lead to, among other things, irritability, mental confusion, and listlessness.

Encouragingly, there appears to be a renewed interest among physicians and scientists today in the importance of nutrition for maintaining an optimum degree of health. And an assessment of the diet of every patient may well become as normal a part of a medical check-up as listening to the heart, taking a urine sample, or checking blood pressure.

Since dance is concerned with the body and with exercise, the dancer should be particularly attentive to a balanced and healthy diet. In this way, dance can lead us into nutritional well-being.

For the dancer, exercise and nutrition work hand in hand. It is essential that the dancer takes an intelligent and disciplined care of the body, giving special attention not just to exercise but to a proper balanced diet. In my experience dancers are notoriously ill-informed about this.

Good health is not simply a matter of what we eat, it is also a matter of how the body converts what we eat into fuel, and this is in part at least dependent upon an efficient and effective physical body system. Normally the system of the dancer's body is in excellent shape, but in the case of non-dancers it may be that here lies another benefit of such an activity as dance.

The therapeutic nature of body contact as related to dance

Dance, as well as being a physical activity, is also a contact activity in that it involves bodily contact with another human being. Included in such contact experiences are touching, embracing, cuddling, holding, leading, carrying, lifting, caressing and pushing. Face to face, hip to hip, and pelvis to pelvis are common formal physical contact expressions within social dance, as are arms around another's waist, shoulders, neck and arm. All these bodily contacts represent legitimate formal codes of social/emotional/physical expression.

For the dance therapist, as well for the ordinary man in the street, this form of expression represents an important source of health and healing. Tactile experiences, used so much in 'self-help groups', 'encounter groups', 'group dynamics' etc, play an important part in dance therapy. One of the characteristic pleasures and motivations for social dance has always been the formal opportunity it provides for human beings, usually of the opposite sex, to relate to each other in a closer intimate/physical and emotional way than usual, but one that is socially acceptable. This has been so throughout the history of social dance. The sort of body contact in social dance is not an end in itself. One does not normally go to a social dance purely for the purpose of having body contact.

One attends for the social, emotional and physical experience it affords, an experience related to another human being in a close way. This joy of sharing and relating through physical contact is marvellously illustrated in such social dance forms as folk dance, national dance, bush dance, square dance, barn dance, and disco dance, to name a few. These events are not frivolous, primitive or disguised erotic entertainments, but rather significant formal structures whereby one is able to relate to another, and by so doing, greatly contribute to one's general well-being. Sadly, these dance expressions are no longer a normal and everyday part of our society, but they do still attract an enormous following in the form of clubs and societies. I read with interest in a daily newspaper here in Western Australia where I am writing:

> Upwards of 4,000 pairs of feet slide into that well-known foxtrot/quickstep formula every week in ballrooms and dance studios throughout Western Australia. Far from killing off interest in ballroom dancing, the disco has contributed to a boom in the more elegant forms of moving the human body to music. More than 50 schools cater for the demand for tuition in the intricacies of the tango, waltz, rumba, samba and cha cha!

K Keating, writing with a cheerful mix of whimsy and profound seriousness in *The Little Book of Hugs*, says:

> Hugging is an instinct, a natural response to feelings of affection, compassion, need and joy. It is also a science, a simple method of support, healing and growth, with immeasurable and remarkable results. Touch is not only nice, it is needed. Research strongly supports the theory that stimulation by touch, in all its forms is necessary for physical, as well as emotional well-being. Hugging feels good, it dispels loneliness, overcomes fears, opens doors to feelings, eases tensions, and affirms our physical being.

> The greatest sense in our body is the sense of touch. We feel, we

love, we hate, are touchy and are 'touched' through the skin.[22]

Touch affects the body's vital forces. It brings energy into the body and allows for its discharge. Some people who lack sufficient body contact are often in direct contact with their anguish in that body tension turns to numbness, coldness, emptiness, frozenness and the feeling of being dead. The body ache and yearning turns into neutrality, and from there into 'stay off'.[23]

Just as dance can be a means of releasing tension in our bodies by vigorous exercise, so, too, can physical contact greatly contribute to easing physical, emotional and social tensions.

Of course, therapy of this sort is not free! The cost is the strength it requires to be vulnerable. The fee for contact is the risk that our 'hugs' will be rebuffed or misinterpreted. Moreover, for many it has fearful implications in that 'some frightened part of us wants to avoid the personal closeness of human intimacy. It is as if the touching has consequences, and we sense that human bonding is brought about by our touching and being touched.'[24] Nevertheless, touching represents a powerful healing potential. When we are prepared to risk reaching out and touching others, we will be free to discover a very real and deep compassion, along with a capacity for joy that exists in all of us. This is bound up with the nature of God who is love and who dwells in each of us. 'As we become more spontaneous and find such inner riches, the fees will soon seem relatively small.'[25]

Sadly, it has to be admitted that body contact is not a norm of our society. This is indicated in an interesting piece of research carried out by S Jourrad into body contact as expressed in the form of touch. While he found that the rate of interpersonal touch in London was nil, in Puerto Rico it was 180 touches per hour![26]

'In Western culture,' writes D J A Edwards, 'the use of touch in interpersonal relationships has, as far as possible, been avoided. Partly because touching infants and children was believed to encourage dependency and weakness, and partly because touching between adults was seen as almost exclusively a sexual matter.'[27]

Bowlby, the famous child psychologist, says much about the effects of tactile deprivation during early childhood and its effects on adulthood: 'The primary and fundamental neglect of touch and body contact is seen today in how we suffer from its lack. Civilisation, in all its institutions and education has failed. . .'

For many years religion especially has played a major role in the control of this powerful area of behaviour:

> It has been one of the great negative achievements of Christianity to make sin of tactile pleasure. Yet this teaching does not arise out of any core teaching of Christianity as such, but out of a failure to make the distinction between touch as a *nutrient* and touch as a *sexual* response.[28]

> *Sexual touch* can be defined as the touching of another person in order to stimulate sexual arousal in one's self or in the person touched. *Nutrient touch* can be defined as the expression of the human capacity for loving and being loved through the body by touching, holding, embracing, stroking, caressing, where sexual arousal is absent, minimal or entirely secondary or marginal.[29]

The taboo on touch which arises out of a failure to discriminate sexual from nutrient touch only perpetuates our blindness to this important distinction, since it rules out the likelihood that anyone will experience touch in adulthood outside the context of a sexual relationship, except perhaps in moments of crisis.

Interestingly, within classical psychoanalysis the relationship between therapist and dis-eased has traditionally been exclusively verbal and touching has been taboo. However, within contemporary research there is a growing support for the powerful healing tool of physical contact, with the result that more counsellors are beginning to make use of this powerful form of human expressions. Touch as a means of healing has been re-evaluated and the place of touch, as a nutrient, is now becoming more fully understood. Edwards writes: 'It is a measure of the individual's development as a human being, the extent to which he or she is freely able to embrace another and enjoy the embrace of others.'[30]

The expression and experience of touch has a wide variety of meanings, both for the one who is touching and the one being touched. It can serve a number of different functions and it is important for the dance therapist to be aware of some of these functions. D J A Edwards has identified nine different types of touch:

> information touch
> prompting touch
> aggressive touch
> nutrient touch
> celebratory touch
> sexual touch
> cathartic touch
> ludic touch

Information touch is that form of touch which is motivated by the need to identify something about the other person, for example, the physiotherapist manipulates a dancer's back to discover the cause of pain.

Prompting touch and movement facilitation touch is that form of touch which is motivated by the need to guide the person physically, for example, a teacher moves the leg of a dancer to indicate the precise nature of the air or floor pattern in an exercise such as a *rond de jambe*.

Aggressive touch is that form of touch which involves

coercion, usually against the other person's will. This type of touch is also used in the dance class, but it is not normally used as punishment but as 'encouragement', and takes the form of a prod, a push, slap or pull.

Nutrient touch is the form of touch that particularly characterises dance and dance therapy. A healer can play a crucial role here in helping the dis-eased to distinguish between sexual and nutrient touch.

Nutrient touch can help someone feel that they belong, that they are secure, accepted, and cared for. It can be a reassurance, comfort and support. It can help the dis-eased person to confront his dis-ease. It can often awaken feelings —physical and emotional—by helping the person learn how to 'give in', to surrender and acknowledge his dis-ease. Getting in touch with the physically and emotionally dis-eased person, and helping them get in touch with themselves, is often a key to the beginning of well-being.

Celebratory touch arises, as the name suggests, out of celebration, out of physical joy and gladness. Joy itself is a great healer, and when it is within the social body and accompanied by human contact it becomes doubly so. How can anyone doubt that if they have ever been part of a social dance evening! As with nutrient touch, celebratory touch represents an essential part of dance as health and healing. 'If we see psychotherapy as being aimed at the teaching of joy, as well as the breaking down of distorted patterns of emotional responding, the celebratory touch has an important place in therapy.'[31]

Sexual touch is motivated by sexual arousal in the other person, and mutual touch is a necessary prelude to sexual intercourse. Heron argues that the most fulfilling sexual intercourse will involve a combination of celebratory, nutrient and even ludic touch to complement the purely sexual. Other writers have argued that inadequate experience of nutrient touch during development can create difficulties in relating sexually in adulthood. From this point of view, then, nutrient touch is not something that arises out of sexual touch, but rather sexual touch needs to be grounded in the nutrient touch. Hence the fundamental importance of nutrient touch.

Cathartic touch is a form of touch designed to help release feelings in the dis-eased. In most cases, for the normal, unhospitalised, dis-eased person the simple act of touching or holding can create an atmosphere of acceptance, and can communicate that your feelings are OK. Body touch therapists use direct touch deliberately to aid emotional arousal, awareness and relief, to break down what Reich called 'body armouring'. Some therapists employ specific manipulations of the body in order to release tension and allow blocked feelings to be released and experienced. As has already been discovered, this can often have the effect of a recovery of repressed memories which then can be worked with therapeutically.

Ludic touch is the sort of touch that occurs in games and sports. In some of the more uninhibited folk dancing there is much ludic touch in the form of back-slapping, 'pig-a-back', 'romp and tumble', bumps, slaps, pushing, shoving, etc. They are all powerful in their therapeutic effect of breaking down social, emotional and physical barriers.

In the dance we see almost all these forms of touching, and legitimately so. This has always been so whether it be expressed in the extreme formality of the eighteenth-century minuet, the uninhibited and somewhat primitive dancing of the disco, or the quiet and polite intimacy of the ballroom. Dance involves ludic, celebratory and nutrient touch especially, but information and prompting touch are also frequently involved. Aggresssive and sexual touch are used much less, and then usually only implicitly in Western society, but they are nevertheless there.

Edwards conducted a piece of research to discover people's

responses to different forms of touch, and especially to the distinction between sexual and nutrient touch. He discovered that the majority of participants in the study found the experience very positive, and that even when touch was experienced as threatening or intrusive, it did not stop it being experienced in a positive way. Clearly, 'the misuse of a good thing should not preclude the possibility of its being a good and lawful thing.'

It is no accident, I believe, that in Jesus' ministry of healing we see again and again the central place of touch. Our Lord was clearly not afraid of physical contact. To touch was a necessary and normal part of healing. 'Jesus reached out his hand and touched the man... Immediately he was cured of his leprosy' (Mt 8:3). 'He took the girl by the hand, and she got up' (Mt 9:25). 'Jesus put his fingers into the man's ears' (Mk 7:33). 'Mary wiped his feet with her hair' (Jn 12:3). These are among the many examples of touching in Jesus' ministry.

> I think back on how Jesus acted while inhabiting a human body on earth. He reached out His hand and touched the eye of the blind, the skin of the person with leprosy, and the legs of the cripple. When the woman pressed against Him in a crowd to tap into the healing energy she hoped he was there, He felt the drain of that energy, stopping the noisy crowd and asking, 'Who touched me?' I have sometimes wondered why Jesus so frequently touched the people He healed, many of whom must have been unattractive, obviously diseased, unsanitary, smelly.[32]

> The way I see it is like this: the Christian shares the life of God himself — that is a certain tenet of Christian belief. The Father, Son and Holy Spirit lives within us. Somehow the energy generated by this life can overflow, can be communicated and flow from one person to another through touching the other person. There is a natural power of life in loving people which is communicated in a special way through the power of touch and

the patient absorbs much of this life energy, in such a way that the sick body can build up its own life building forces.[33]

Relaxation

Relaxation is here meant to refer to 'the capacity to release muscular tension from whatever cause it is derived—physical, mental, emotional or social—and to adjust effort in amount and sequence for a smooth efficient functioning of all aspects of human well-being.' There is in most of us a great need for deep rest and freedom from the unrelenting stress and strain that seems to characterise Western society today. And this is as much a problem, if not more of a problem, for the Christian. As Christians we are supposed to seek our peace *through* the faith and yet a paradox frequently exists where the seeking of that peace produces its own tensions. 'There is a pervasive form of contemporary violence to which the [Christian] idealist, fighting for peace by non-violent methods, most easily succumbs: activism and overwork.'[34] The rush and pressure of modern life are a form, perhaps the most common form, of innate violence. Is this you? It has certainly been me, I am ashamed to say.

> To allow oneself to be carried away by a multitude of conflicting concerns, to surrender to too many demands, to commit oneself to too many projects, to want to help everyone in everything, is to succumb to violence. More than than, it is a co-operation with violence. The frenzy of the activist neutralises his work for peace. It destroys his inner capacity for peace.[35]

I am reminded that Elijah on Mount Horeb was looking for God in the thunder of earthquake, fire and lightning. But he found his God in 'the still small voice'. In a world which seems so void of stillness and silence we need to create stillness and silence, where we can begin to get in touch with the more cosmic and spiritual dimensions of our human being. Dance, as with music, can contribute uniquely and profoundly to this inner dimension.

It is important to recognise that relaxation is of supreme importance to health and healing. The first impulse on feeling pain is to stop moving and thus tighten up. In this state of tension the muscles contract, constricting the blood flow and causing swelling as more circulation is cut off. This leads to a vicious circle: more pain, more tightening, more stiffness, more swelling. This circle can be broken if you begin to relax in body, mind and heart. Fresh blood then begins to bring nourishment to the afflicted areas and healing can begin.

On one level, relaxation may be experienced through the dance technique class. And one of the simplest methods is the progressive letting go and relaxing of major muscle groups from the feet to the head. The dance teacher quietly and carefully guides the dis-eased through a progressive awareness of his or her body, making sure that in every case the body begins to 'let go' and relaxes until the whole is at rest. This is usually done at the beginning of a class, while lying on the ground, but in my experience it is particularly beneficial when it is done on the completion of a technique class, when the body has been exercised vigorously and the muscles have been relieved of their blocked energy, and when there is a general sense of well-being, and a need to relax following such strenuous exercise.

Relaxation, surprisingly, produces relief in a wide variety of stress-related symptoms including tension and migraine head-aches, chronic pain symptoms of all types, functional gastro-intestinal disturbances, atropic symptoms including hay fever, eczma and asthma; mild hypertension, menstrual disfunction; and symptoms directly attributable to anxiety. Given the per-suasive influence of stress and tension in medical and psychiatric patients and in the 'worried well' in modern society it may seem that relaxational skills should be something we should all learn as an essential part of preventative medicine.[36]

Relaxation and dance

The search for inner peace, which we all make, is as much the concern of the 'outer' body as it is of the 'inner'. Both affect each other. One of the major elements of health and healing not normally associated with the dance is that of peace and relaxation, of stillness rather than motion. Dance is seen mainly in terms of victorious joyful and celebratory actions and, indeed, this is essentially the description of dance we see in Scripture where it is synonymous with joy, gladness, happiness and well-being, and is frequently contrasted with mourning. As today, dance in the Bible times was not normally associated with relaxation, with peace and calm; yet it is certainly there. If one thinks of the great classical adagios in ballet, the grand pas de deux from Act 2 of Swan Lake, for example, do we not experience something of ineffable peace arising from tranquility and beauty, and are we not refreshed by the experience? Similarly, within the folk dance tradition there are many dances which are not concerned with the exuberant and joyful, but are more focused on the quiet and meditative. This is perhaps particularly so of our Eastern neighbours. Within the relatively recent tradition of liturgical dance as expressed in the work of such companies as Cedar Dance Theatre, The Sacred Dance, Springs Dance Company and Christian Dance Ministries, place is certainly given to the quiet spiritual and meditative. Those of you who have experienced some of the dances outlined in *Time to Dance* (Collins: London, 1984) or *Dance and the Christian Faith* (Hodder and Stoughton: London, 1985) or have listened to the music of Taizé, for example, 'Adoramus te Domine', 'Veni Creator Spiritus', and 'Ostende nobis', will recognise something of the more meditative and spiritual aspects of the dance. Two well-known contemporary spiritual songs, 'Father we adore you' and 'There's a quiet understanding', are designed to bring about a relaxed meditative response from the worshipper.

So, having begun to master the importance of basic physical relaxation through the technique class we can now begin to experience the peace that comes through the dance itself, involving mind, heart and body. In its meditative form, dance represents a special form of relaxation. All too often with the predominantly youthful church dance group the more meditative and impressionistic aspect of dance is neglected. But dance is often at its most profound and spiritual when it is meditative.

As the body, and the mind and the heart relax, so we begin to open ourselves to the working of the Holy Spirit. There is a growing sense of deep inner peace, a peace that is beyond man's understanding.

> The full meditative experience is beyond the relaxation of the body and mind, beyond the transcendence of discomfort— expect the experience of a deep naturalness, utter naturalness. It is only when this comes to us that we realise that true naturalness is something quite foreign to us in our ordinary lives. Simplicity, such profound simplicity that we are almost overwhelmed by it, immersed in it.[37]

Christian meditation brings with it a profound peace of mind because it dwells upon Jesus, the originator and restorer of peace. It focuses more on listening than speaking, on impressions rather than expressions, on the inner rather than the outer, on the Creator rather than the creature.

Notes

1. Paul Brand and Philip Yancey, *Fearfully and Wonderfully Made* (Hodder and Stoughton: London).

2. Phillip Keller, *Walking with God* (Kingsway: Eastbourne, 1982).

3. Thomas Merton, *Conjectures of a Bystander* (Doubleday Image: London, 1968).

4. C S Lewis, *The Four Loves* (Fontana: London, 1963).

5. Leslie Weatherhead, *Psychology, Religion and Health* (A James).

6. Howard Marshall, *Renewal and Worship*.

7. Thomas Merton, *op cit*.

8. J M Brown Ed, *Vision of Modern Dance* (Dance Books: London).

9. 'The Medical Forum', article in *Harvard Medical School Health Letter* vol 10, no 5 (April, 1985).

10. M Bricklin, *Natural Health and Healing* (Rodale, 1983).

11. Elizabeth Lerman, article in *The Journal of Physical Education, Recreation and Dance* (January, 1986).

12. Selwyn Hughes, *God Wants You Whole* (Kingsway: Eastbourne, 1984).

13. Alexander Lowen, *Betrayal of the Body* (Collier MacMillan: West Drayton, 1969).

14. W Reich, *Character Analysis* (Farrar, Strauss and Giroux).

15. E Rosen, *Dance and Psychotherapy* (Dance Horizons, 1974).

16. R Eide, 'The Effect of Physical Activity on Emotional Reactions, Stress Reactions and Related Physiological Reactions', *Scandinavian Journal of Social Medicine* Supplement 29.

17. S Awaki, 'An Assessment of dance therapy to improve retarded adult body image', *Perc. Motor Skills* 43:2, December 1976.

18. R Eide, 'The Relationship Between Body Image, Self Image and Physical Activity', *Scandinavian Journal of Social Medicine* Supplement 29.

19. G Boryensko, 'Emotions and Your Health', *Vogue* November 1982.

20. B Strickland and K Kendall Psychological Symptoms: the Importance of Assessing Health Status. *Clinical Psychological Review* vol 3.3(2) 1983.

21. W B Saunders, *Health* (Byrd 1961).

22. Paul Brand and Philip Yancey, *op cit*.

23. J Liss, *Free to Feel* Wildwood House.

24. J Powell, *Will the Real Me Stand Up?* Argus Comm. 1985.

25. K Keating, *The Little Book of Hugs*.

26. S Jourrad in *The Observer*, 5th June 1983.
27. J A Edwards, 'The Role of Touch in interpersonal relations; implications for Psychotherapy', *South African Journal of Psychotherapy* 1981.
28. J A Edwards, *ibid.*
29. J. Heron, *Catharsis in Human Development*, British Post Graduate Medical Federation 1977.
30. J A Edwards, *op cit.*
31. J A Edwards, *op cit.*
32. Paul Brand and Philip Yancey, *op cit.*
33. Frances MacNutt, *The Power to Heal*, Ave Maria Press, 1977.
34. Thomas Merton, *op cit.*
35. Thomas Merton, *op cit.*
36. A A Sheik, ed. *Imagination and Healing*, Baywood Press, 1984.
37. H Benson, *The Relaxation Response*, Fount, 1975.

5

The Emotional Dimension of Human Being

Scripture and emotional health

The feeling, or heartfelt aspect of our human being, is important to a proper understanding of God. It is through our hearts that the Holy Spirit pours God's love (Rom 5:5). In Scripture the word 'heart' usually refers to our innermost being, where decisions are made and actions issue forth. In a properly orientated person, this will mean that our feelings are affected by those decisions and by our apprehension of the truth. The New Testament Church is built not on tablets of stone, but human hearts (2 Cor 3:3), whereas Jesus had found that all too often people worshipped with their lips, but their hearts were far from him (Mk 7:6). As important as the written word most certainly is, by itself it does not lead to wholeness and a true and full knowledge and understanding of our being and of God. It is with our hearts that we believe. We are commanded to love the Lord with all our hearts, as well as mind.

Whilst 'everything God created is good, and nothing is to be rejected if it is received with thanksgiving' (1 Tim 4:4) we do have to recognise that the freedom God in his love allows us, can sometimes separate us from him (Is 59:2). The heart, of all dimensions of our human be-ing, is the most fallible. As Jeremiah warns, 'The heart is deceitful above all things and beyond cure. Who can understand it?' (Jer 17:9). Things that come out of our mouths usually issue forth from a deceitful heart, and it is these feelings and thoughts that make us unclean. 'What comes out of a man is what makes him "unclean". For from within, out of men's hearts, come evil thoughts, sexual immorality, theft, murder, adultery, greed, malice, deceit, lewdness, envy, slander, arrogance and folly. All these evils come from inside and make a man "unclean"' (Mk 7:20−22). 'However, a man can bring good things out of the good that is stored up in his heart, out of the overflow of his heart his mouth also speaks' (Lk 6:45). In these two scriptural passages we see something of the twofold, paradoxical nature of our heart and feelings. 'When our hearts are rooted in the word then our eyes, feelings, bodies and everyday actions will be full of light. But when they are not, they will be bad and full of darkness' (Lk 11:34).

Since a person sees God through the eyes of the heart, 'Blessed are the pure in heart' (Mt 5:8). Without this pure heart we will not see God. In order that our hearts may be right with God we need to be 'transformed by the renewing of our minds' (Rom 12:2). As we think with our minds, so will we feel in our hearts. As we both think and feel, so we will act. The mind, we are reminded yet again, is of fundamental importance to a pure heart. The heart, or feeling nature of our human being is God given and originally good, it is essential to health and wholeness, but it must be rooted in the written word.

In order that we may become as our Creator would have us be, in order to be healthy and whole, and free of emotional disease let us be rid of 'sexual immorality, impurity and debauchery, idolatry and witchcraft; hatred, discord, jealousy, fits of rage, selfish ambition, dissensions, factions and envy; drunkenness, orgies, and the like' (Gal 5:19−21). 'Malice and deceit, hypocrisy, envy and slander of every kind' (1 Pet 2:1). Instead we are to clothe ourselves with 'compassion, kindness, humility, gentleness and patience. Bear with each other and forgive whatever grievances you may have against one another' (Col 3:12–13), for the fruit of the Spirit is 'love, joy, peace, patience, kindness, goodness, faithfulness, gentleness and self control' (Gal 5:22). Love is patient, kind, rejoices in the truth, protects, trusts, hopes and perseveres. It does not boast, it is not proud, rude, self seeking, and easily angered, it does not keep a record of wrongs and does not delight in evil (1 Cor 13:4–7).

A diseased heart, a heart which is ill at ease, is very often the consequence of a diseased mind. Emotional health is dependent upon a faithful obedience to God's laws as laid down in Scripture. Health and healing of emotional disease involve an adherence to Jesus Christ, a complete dependence on him and obedience to him.

In order to be freed from emotional disease we must acknowledge our sins before God. 'If we confess our sins, he is faithful and just and will forgive us our sins and purify us from all unrighteousness' (1 Jn 1:9). But if we keep silent about our sins, our bones will waste away through our groaning all day long (Ps 32:3). And indeed 'the whole creation has been groaning as in the pains of childbirth right up to the present time' (Rom 8:22). Every human being from the beginning of time, and including the spiritual giants as recorded in the Bible like Jonah, Elijah, Jeremiah, Moses, Naomi, Peter, and Paul, all experienced sickness in many forms, including emotional disease. It was partly for this reason that God sent Jesus: to disarm the principalities and powers and make a public spectacle of them, triumphing over them by the cross (Col 2:15). 'He came that we might have life, and have it to the full' (Jn 10:10). As we seek the truth so will we be set free from our disease.

Moreover 'we do not have a high priest who is unable to sympathise with our weaknesses, but we have one who has been tempted in every way, just as we are—yet was without sin' (Heb 4:15). So when our hearts *are* overwhelmed, we can return to your rock that is higher than we are (Ps 61:2). All the weary and burdened—the diseased in mind, body, heart and spirit—can come to him for rest (Mt 11:28).

Emotionally diseased we are encouraged to come to him, *as we are,* in the full assurance of faith that he will forgive and restore us. But we must come honestly and wholeheartedly, and in faith. There can be no healing until we want to be healed, whatever our condition! A broken and contrite heart, certainly, he will not despise, for 'the sacrifices of God *are* a broken spirit' (Ps 51:17). They are a prerequisite for health and healing.

Let us ask that he create in us a clean *heart* and a renewed spirit (Ps 51:10).

'There is a time to weep and a time to laugh, a time to mourn and a time to dance' (Eccles 3:4). That is the nature of life, and of man, and especially his emotional life. God's hand is in it all. But even through our emotional ups and downs we are exhorted to *rejoice* in the Lord always (Phil 4:4). This shows that rejoicing can be an act of the will that, when necessary, will override the emotions, and prove to us that the joy of the Lord is our strength (Neh 8:10).

Emotions and health

God created us in his own image. He endowed us with the capacity to experience and to express feelings and emotions. They are, therefore, a legitimate part of human be-ing. They should be seen, first of all, as something good, bestowed upon us by our heavenly Father to enrich our lives and the lives of those around us. We should not be ashamed of our feelings, however naked they may be. While human emotions may become distorted and misused because of the fallen nature of man, this should not lead us to conclude that the end of our spiritual life is the suppression of our feelings—it is rather their transfiguration. Let us not forget that Jesus Christ, having taken on our nature, has sanctified all our actions, all our feelings.

To affirm our emotions is not to affirm emotionalism, as is so often feared by the church. I recognise only too well the weakness of this position. As David Watson points out:

Concentrating on the purely subjective side of the Christian faith, of feelings of love and joy, peace etc, is but one step away from confusion, deception, agnosticism and even atheism. The Jesus trip in the sixties was for many thousands of young people very attractive emotionally during their spiritual honeymoon period. But when the battles and trials came, the subjective ('sand') experiences began to fade and there was no objective historical ('rock') foundation to fall back on. [1]

Christian love is not blind. Heart, emotions and mind must work together so that we have both a 'discerning love' and a 'loving discernment'. When our feelings are the product of our faith rather than the source of our faith, they will assume a rightful place in the Christian experience. Just as wrong thoughts can seriously influence and undermine a healthy mind so, too, can wrong feelings seriously influence and undermine a healthy 'heart', causing sickness and disease. In both cases there is a need for an underpinning of the word of God.

J B Philips writes:

English people are unfairly suspicious of their emotions. We link emotion with the sentimental, the weak and the unmanly and it has become second nature to us to repress outward signs of emotions.

However desirable that maybe as a national trait, it is silly to act as if reason was a thing to be trusted and the emotions were purely a set of savage animals to be kept under strict control! For all that happens is that emotions which are never recognised remain undeveloped and distrusted. If, on the other hand, they are frankly recognised as the great driving force of life, without there having necessarily to be any outward display of 'emotionalism', our lives will be fuller and richer.[2]

Our emotions can be trained just as our minds can be trained. Unfortunately, we seem to spend years training our minds but spend very little time on training our emotions.

For some strange reason, even though he admits that his personality is made up of thinking, willing and feeling, man, although proud of the thinking that has led him to the system of philosophy and to scientific invention, proud also of achievement of the human will, is ashamed of his emotions. Emotion is the 'poor relation' of personality.[3]

Many Christians are taught to control or repress their feelings and that somehow feelings and emotions are sinful and priority should be given to the mind and will. While it is true that our emotions need to be transformed and guided by the Spirit of God in the written word, 'we must also recognise, in humility and faith, that certain desires and certain pleasures are willed for us by God. We cannot live in truth if we automatically suspect all desires and all pleasures. It is humility to accept our humanity, and pride to reject it. It is simply not *practical,* it is not *honest,* it is not *Christian* to fly from every desire and every pleasure that is not explicitly pious.'[4] Let us accept in faith all our feelings and praise God for them.

A sad and cruel sin is holding back feelings for another — we may say we love someone, but in reality out hearts may be far from him. One of the most tragic effects of misguided religious teaching is the witholding of affection for another rising out of a misplaced piety, a fear of dangerous emotions. Sterility results from a misplaced emphasis on theological abstractions and the priority of the mind, and a code of conduct is laid down that emotions are not compatible with mature Christian faith and can lead us very easily into sin. As G K Chesterton once said, 'The meanest fear is fear of sentimentality. It would add immeasurably to the amount of love abroad if we would be freer in declaring our affection. Jesus had a way of doing it. He declared in a hundred different ways that He loved.' The healing power of love and affection is extremely powerful as we shall see shortly. Conversely, one of the most powerful single sources of disease is the absence or withdrawal of love and affection. It lies at the root of many of our diseases. Is it any wonder that the first two commandments are described as the most important of all commandments and upon which all other commandments are based?

The fact is, many of us have allowed ourselves to be squeezed into the mould of worldly thinking. We need to have our minds renewed and transformed. We have denied ourselves the richness of emotional experience and expression that Christian living and worshipping entails. If anyone should doubt the legitimacy of feelings and emotional expression as an essential part of human being, let him study the Psalms. Even a cursory glance will not fail to convince him that such healthy and uninhibited expressions were considered normal and lawful, from the 'mourning' end of the continuum to the 'dancing'. We see anger, wrath, tears, gnashing of teeth, being consumed by anguish, wailing and beseeching, as well as dancing, shouting in praise, clapping, rejoicing, being glad, singing in joy, and laughing. 'In the service of God there is perfect freedom; we come as we are, we can be ourselves without fear or shame, or the need for justification when we give of ourselves in child-like faith to Him. He accepts us as we are.'[4]

Faith is primarily an intellectual assent. But if it were only that and nothing more, it would not be complete. It has to be something more than an assent of the mind, it must include our hearts (Mk 7:6; 2 Cor 3:3).

One of the causes of emotional disease is this exclusiveness of the intellect as expressed in propositional knowledge, and the neglect of the heart. Language is, of course, a primary and public instrument of expression, and it is significant that even in non-verbal therapy most psychotherapists acknowledge the view that ultimately there must be concern for verbal or intellectual articulation for any real and lasting healing to take place. But it is also being increasingly recognised that an important part of reality is quite inaccessible to such language. And this is where the non-verbal expressive art therapies come in. 'The primary function of art,' argues Susan Langer, dance philosopher, 'is to objectify feelings so we can contemplate and understand them, the formulation of so-called inward experience, "the inner life", that is impossible to achieve by discursive thought—the life of feeling is not irrational, its logical forms are merely very different from the structures of discourse. What discursive symbols—language in the literal sense— does for our awareness of things about us, and our own relation to them, the arts do for our awareness of subjective reality, feeling and emotion.'[5]

It has been estimated that the root cause of something like three-quarters of most physical disease is rooted in the heart and mind rather than the body. Psychosomatic medicine is not a twentieth-century discovery but a rediscovery of well-established, ancient biblical truths (see Psalms 32 and 38). It is not emotion in itself that causes physical disease in the body, but rather its supression and the armouring and defence against it. Much disease is the consequence of unresolved, unexpressed needs and emotional states. By unexpressed needs I do not mean exclusively negative emotions such as fear, anger, grief, bitterness and resentments. Supression of such feelings and expression as love, joy and creativity can also bring about sickness and disease. It is a sobering and somewhat disturbing thought that because of our fears and inhibitions about our feelings and affections, and especially our feelings and affections for each other, we may, by denying the expression of God's love which is in each of us and is designed for us (1 Jn 4:7–12), be inadvertently contributing to sickness and disease.

John Powell writes:

> Very often such needs cannot be acknowledged or expressed. They do not coincide, for example, with the image of independent virility that is thrust upon us by society and culture, consequently, the person who is forced to repress these needs has to seek his gratification elsewhere, and usually in devious and subtle ways at times, sadly and even tragically, deceiving himself.[6]

Psychosomatic medicine declares that the negative effects of emotions cannot be indulged in for any length of time without eventually some unwholesome effect upon the body. The strongest steel breaks if kept too long under unrelieved tension. Inner emotions must be released. Repression takes a terrible toll, and is the source of some of our most troublesome physical problems.

In the same way that mental honesty is essential for mental health, so, too, is emotional honesty essential to emotional health. Fundamental to honesty, authenticity and truth—all intimately related as we have seen from Scripture—is confession. There can be no healing from within until there is confession without. Confessing is essential to cleansing. (See Psalm 32 especially for a very explicit statement about unconfessed sin and its responsibility for physical, mental and emotional disease.)

The concept of confession I have in mind involves a broader and more basic range of truth and honesty than is traditional within the church. It is concerned with something much more than admitting outward misbehaviours. It is based

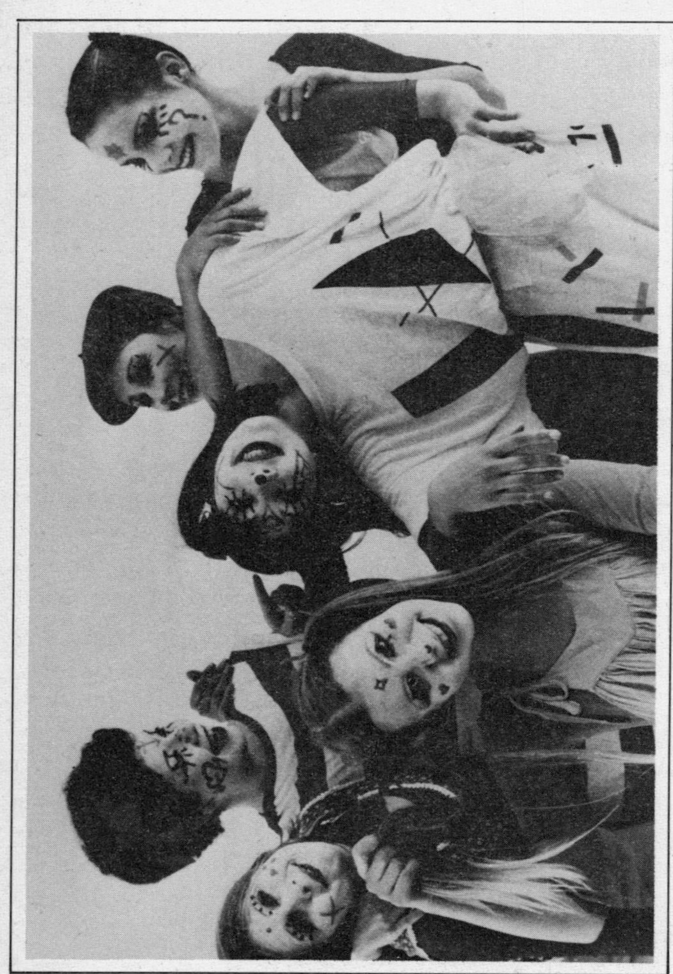

'How good and pleasant it is when brothers live in unity! For there the Lord bestows his blessing, even life for evermore' (Ps 133).

rather on an underlying truth: that of 'authenticity' and 'individuation', ourselves as we really are, good or bad! Within the context of emotional being, this entails an open and honest admittance to everything that goes to make up this aspect of our life, irrespective of whether or not it is good or bad. It is a confessing and opening up in loving obedience believing, in faith, that this is the key to health and healing. When our consciousness is blocked, we can neither face ourselves nor the world around us. Until we have opened ourselves to God in humble confession, the blockage and the disease caused by it will remain. Unless we can come as we are, we cannot be-come. Until one is right with oneself, the healing powers cannot be fully put into effect.

One cannot live with the lie, the untrue, no matter how 'good' it is. Acknowledging what is, provides a real and honest base from which to be healed, restored and forgiven. On the other hand, a lie gnaws at the centre of our being, it blocks spontaneity and destroys the integrative quality of the self. It leads to self-deception and self-negation. When we resort to acting or wearing masks, there is no possibility of true growth. It is only when we are able to face the naked truth about ourselves that we are able to begin to experience any kind of liberation and healing.

Acknowledging the truth about ourselves is often painful.

The man is perfect in faith who can come to God in the utter dearth of his feelings, and desires, without a glow or an inspiration, with the weight of low thoughts, failures, neglects and wondering forgetfulness and say to Him, 'Thou art my refuge'.[7]

The function of dance and movement therapy as it relates to emotional health and healing is basically twofold.

First, to facilitate through the discipline and the non-verbal language of dance and movement a means of releasing and relieving emotional dis-eases which arise from unresolved and unexpressed emotional states. This function is essentially 'cathartic' and 'symptomatic'. Secondly, to provide a formal disciplined means whereby the dis-eased is able to (a) *experience* emotions and feelings and (b) *express* emotions and feelings, ie, initiating his or her own inner feeling life through the language of dance. This function is essentially 'educational' and 'symbolic'.

Dance in both cases represents a means whereby emotional expression either in the predominantly 'symptomatic' form of the first or the more 'symbolic' form of the second, is attained.

Dance and emotional health

To talk about 'blocked energy', energy being 'dammed up', energy being 'released', 'cleared' or 'broken down' is the language of body therapy work. It is also part of the language of dance therapy.

The idea of 'working off' and releasing body energies resulting from anger, frustrations and indignations etc by involving oneself in vigorous physical activity has long since been recognised as an efficient and effective way of 'letting off steam' or releasing emotional tension. This principle of 'letting off steam' lies at the root of all body and dance therapy.

When feelings are 'blocked', for whatever reason, conscious or unconscious, the body is unable to externalise what is being felt. When the feelings of our inner life continue to send messages to the body and the body cannot act on impulse the result, eventually, is an overworked circuit. One of the primary concerns of dance therapy is with the releasing of such blocked and buried feelings. This unblocking, as already indicated, takes two forms: 'symptomatic' movement expression and 'symbolic' movement expression.

In 'symptomatic' expression the dis-eased is encouraged to give vent to his feelings in an essentially unthinking, spontaneous and intuitive way. The emphasis here is on encouraging an open, honest and uninhibited expression. This expression will reflect the physical and mental state we are in and the emotions that stir us. 'It is possible that the therapeutic agent here is similar to the therapeutic function of dreams, that of, as it were, bypassing consciousness, in the sense that both are created by the spontaneous overflow of powerful feelings, both generate an archaic content, both produce a reprieve from reality, an occasional suspension of the inner trial and the inner disbelief.'[8]

In 'symbolic' expression, which has its roots in 'symptomatic' expression, the dis-eased is encouraged to work at a more conscious, deliberate and formal, artistic level. Here the emphasis is less on catharsis, in the primitive sense at least, and more on 'education' and 'integration'. Symptomatic expression stirs the contents of the unconscious and encourages it to move into the conscious, thus promoting the process of understanding and integration. The dis-eased is encouraged to realise and express what has become conscious at a more 'symbolic' level—through the dance. Symbolic expression extends and refines our knowledge, taking us beyond the scope of actual experience. It is more 'presentational' than 'representational' in that it goes beyond what is. Dance as therapy then, is both 'symptomatic' and 'symbolic', 'representational' and 'presentational'.

In dance therapy the dis-eased is provided with a formal channel through which he or she can project the inner self, and thus begin to release tensions built up as a result of negative emotional reaction. Self-expression in this sense of the term, usually abhorrent to the dance artist, is positively encouraged in dance as therapy and may well involve the dis-eased person 'expressing himself all over the floor' in a free, spontaneous and uninhibited way. As the repressed or denied feelings come to the surface and move from the unconscious into the conscious, the dis-eased not only feels a great physical and emotional release from the tension, but also begins to understand at a more symbolic, non-verbal level something of the nature of the dis-ease. Unless the individual is able to reach himself at this root level there can be no proper and lasting healing.

One of the first steps in dance as therapy is to try to make contact with the unconscious and sub-conscious, with the repressed and suppressed aspects of human being. One way of doing this is by 'becoming' what we have renounced or suppressed, in order that we can be released from what 'blocks' us. In the cathartic experience we must first acknowledge our hurts and anguish, and then be prepared to relive them by making 'outward' what has been 'inward'. In the case of depression, where anger is characteristically directed inward, the diseased is encouraged to actualise and make concrete the buried feelings. Learning to be angry is a necessary task for most of us hurt by our own feelings. The same process holds true for emotions like grief, loss, rejection, resentment and bitterness. All emotional effects withheld and frozen within the body have to be acknowledged and released in outward physical and emotional terms. Bioenergetic exercises — which are the hallmark of Alexander Lowens' work in body therapy — stamping, punching, kicking, shouting, are all important steps in the process of 'taking the heat' out of self-hurt. Stuck feelings must be permitted to undergo a period of intensification for there to be release. A stuck emotional reaction implies that there was no opportunity for awareness and expression. The feeling, stifled in its expression and held back from consciousness, is not discharged, with the result that the undischarged emotional energy produces untoward symptoms: tension, pain, agitation, frustration and general overall pre-occupation with unlocatable distress.

This identification and expression of repressed and suppressed feelings must take place within the context of self-control which is, after all, one of the fruits of God's Spirit within us.

Thought patterns produce feelings, and feelings produce actions. Therefore, any permanent reduction in dis-ease must deal with the problems of thought patterns. Cathartic release, although of primary importance, is only a short-term expedient and symptomatic expression. Most therapists would agree that physical release greatly helps the patient to be more open to a higher form of therapy, one that includes the mind through public forms of communication. In the later stages of healing it is generally agreed that movement and cognitive work should be viewed as complementary. Thus, once again, reinforcing as in Scripture, the primacy of the word. As one therapist puts it: 'Mere spontaneous outbursts, the mere loosening up or letting go, is as incomplete a performance artistically as it is humanly.'9 Another therapist writes: 'The release of energy itself is of questionable value. Energy without form can grow more evil, while evil in a recognised shape can be met and dealt with in some way. What is unconscious cannot be modified or educated until it is made conscious.'

Dance therapy is not only concerned with catharsis, the process of releasing and acting out one's inner hurts. Its ultimate and aim is education, the development of an active, responsible knowledge and understanding of one's emotional life. It is concerned with providing clear, formal, disciplined avenues of consciousness through which the individual can both experience and express the inner feelings of his human being. By 'experience', I refer to the willingness and ability actually to feel emotion. And by 'expression', I refer to the ability to identify and articulate emotion. These are essentially two sides of the same coin. Emotional problems, in my experience, are as much to do with what people do not or cannot feel as they are to do with what they do and can. Emotional health depends, first of all, on being emotionally authentic. This is one dimension of personality we dare not deny. When our emotional life is acknowledged and accepted for what it is, we can always educate, correct and extend, as the case may be. But if we refuse to acknowledge and accept our inner life as it is, there will be no true long-term healing.

'Symbolic' movement expression, a deliberate and conscious emotional act, is the eventual concern of dance health and healing. It is concerned with a concept of art as the creation of perceptible forms expressive of human feeling. Susan Langer comments:

> Feeling covers much more than it does in the technical vocabulary of psychology. It takes in all possible meanings: it applies to *everything* that can be felt. The word expression has two principle meanings: in one sense it means self-expression, giving vent to one's feelings. In this sense it refers to a symptom of what we feel. In another sense, however, it means presentation of an idea in the symbolic perceptible sense of the term.[10]

Dance, in this symbolic sense of the term, includes a wide variety of movement expressions, all of which can provide 'impressions' and 'expressions' of feeling and emotion. The responsibility of the dance therapist is to identify the particular needs of the therapy group, and then select the dance forms appropriate for the realisation of such needs. Among these dance forms are ballet, ballroom, jazz, tap, aerobics, historic, national and folk, ethnic, modern, and religious dance. No dance form can be specifically identified as therapeutic. In the sense that all dance forms contribute to therapy, they are all therapeutic. But having said that, I would add that there is, perhaps, one particular dance expression that more than any other in my experience is especially conducive to dance therapy, and that is 'creative dance'. In creative dance, as opposed to most other forms of dance, the dancer is both the creator and performer. He originates the choreography and interprets that creation in action. In both cases the creature is the creator and creation. His instrument of expression, his medium of expression, and the expression itself all originate from the unique individual. There is no other dance form quite like this. This is not to imply, of course, that in the more choreographed dances there is no place for individual creation. And movement does not by itself equal the dance experience. The dancer always has to invest something of his or herself in a pattern or sequence of movements, whatever form that dance may take. In doing so he is being creative, or more accurately, interpretive or recreative. These dance expressions, although imposed from without, are particularly beneficial in the impressionistic sense of the term expression. Since they come from without and are imposed upon the dancer, they provide invaluable experiences that are not of the individual and which therefore extend and refine that individual's experience of both dance and expression.

But creative dance, I must emphasise, is not mere uninhibited hip-swinging! Creative dance, in the symbolic sense of the term, involves a disciplined, skilful concern for at least three prerequisites:

(1) The *instrument* of expression — the body.
(2) The *medium* of expression — movement.
(3) The *art* and *craft* of expression — the skill of composition and expression.

(For a more detailed critical discussion of the importance of creative dance skill, see *Dance and the Christian Faith*.)

Celebration

'A cheerful heart is good medicine' (Prov 17:22).

A brief word about the traditionally predominant celebratory aspect of dance as it relates to health and healing.

The way of the cross is sometimes painful and brings with it much hurt and suffering as we learn to love — ourselves, each other, and God. This is a normal and 'healthy' part of Christian growth. There is 'a time to weep and a time to laugh, a time to mourn and a time to dance' (Eccles 3:4). God's desire is not to ignore nor sometimes even to eradicate pain and suffering, but rather to transform it.

In the same way as such negative feelings as bitterness, resentment, anger and depression can contribute to emotional disease, so too can positive feelings of happiness, joy, gladness and making merry contribute towards emotional well-being. Celebration can be an effective antidote for the sense of sadness that sometimes oppresses the heart. Just as tears can be a release from tension, so can laughter. Tears and laughter are often very close, as C S Lewis wrote: 'There is a peculiar quality of joy that only comes through pain. There is a certain intensity and brilliance of joy that is only experienced through suffering and pain.'[11] Perhaps that is why we are commanded to 'rejoice in the Lord always' (Phil 4:4).

Praising God is surely one of the most effective spiritual therapies for the depressed Christian. Perhaps the most positive thing that comes out of such celebration, even when we are not in the mood for it, is that it decentralises self. Being diseased sometimes makes it very difficult to get outside of oneself. 'In the celebratory dance we see a shift of centre from self to God. One cannot praise God without relinquishing occupation with self. Praise produces forgetfulness of self—and a forgetfulness of self is health.'[12] The Psalmist's injunction to 'delight yourself in the Lord' (Ps 37:4) is a specific instruction for us to follow, and for good healthy reasons. No fewer than forty-one of the Psalms specifically refer to 'singing praises unto God'. As Richard Foster says:

Celebration is at the heart of the way of Christ. He entered the world on a high note of jubilation: 'I bring you good news of great joy,' cried the angel, 'which shall come to all the people' (Lk 2:10), and He left the world bequeathing His joy to the disciples: 'I have told you this so that my joy may be in you, and that joy may be complete' (Jn 15:11).[13]

Celebration brings joy and 'dancing' into our life; and this makes us strong. Scripture tells us that the joy of the Lord *is* our strength (Neh 8:10). It is one of the fruits of the Spirit (Gal 5:22). Did you know that laughter apparently triggers off endozymes that are natural morphone—like pain-killers? As Proverbs 17:22 says, 'A cheerful heart is good medicine, but a crushed spirit dries up the bones.'

Dance throughout Scripture, both in literal and metaphorical terms, is synonymous with celebration, praise and thanksgiving. 'Rejoicing', 'feasting' and 'music-making' by definition imply an intimate association with the dance. Scripture urges us to offer sacrifices of praise to God continually, 'the fruit of lips that confess his name' (Heb 13:15).

Once again, let us see what the pioneers of early modern dance say about emotional expression and dance:
Louis Fuller writes:

> Surprise, deception, content, uncertainty, resignation, hope, distress, joy, fatigue, feebleness and finally death. Are not all these sensations, each in turn, humanity's lot? And why cannot these things be expressed by the dance, guided intelligently, as well as by life itself?

Ruth St Dennis writes:

> The word dancer should rightly mean one who expresses in bodily gesture the joy and power of his being. I see them [dancers] giving praise; praise for the earth and the sky and the sea and the hills, in free, happy movements that are projections of their moods of peace and adoration.

Virginia Stewart writes:

> The modern dance springs out of the very heart of man. It goes back to the source of human life. It throws away superficiality and moves out into the open spaces where abide the heart and soul of mankind.

Martha Graham writes:

> The reality of the dance is its truth to our inner life. Therein lies its power to move and communicate.
>
> The dance always remains bound by the human body, which is after all, the dancer's instrument. However, with the emotion which stirs him and the spirituality which uplifts him, the dance becomes more than mere physical movement in space, and the dancer more than its mobile agent. From then on, it represents the internal experiences of the dancer. From the crudest reality to the sublimest abstraction, man is personified in the dance. All his struggles, griefs, joys are thus represented.[14]

Music and dance — music as therapy

A brief word about music as it relates to the healing process of the emotions seems appropriate here. I have said very little about music so far, except to say that, along with drama, it is intimately related to dance. It seems to me that almost everything I have said about dance can be legitimately applied to music. The only difference being the means or 'language' of expression. In dance therapy a careful consideration of music, as well as drama, is essential.

Psychologists have studied the effect made on the group by different types of music. It was observed, for example, that 'serious contemporary' music, probably less familiar than classical or popular, helped inhibited patients to bring repressed emotions into consciousness. It was also found that romantic music does not always help group integrations, since it tends to arouse personal associations and creates tension, but classical music seemed to help towards the cohesion of the group because of the sense of security it aroused. Traditional music and folk songs were by far the most effective way of bringing together and integrating the group because of their deep-seated and cosmic relationship.[15]

Dr Sydney Mitchell has observed that impressionist music, that is music of a sensuous, fluid character, enables the listener to drift along with the music and gives greater opportunities for deep-seated ideas to come to the surface. He observed that it is often the dreamy, non-emotional, sensuous quality of music that penetrates without provoking the patients' resistance to more potent music. Moreover, sensuous melodic music has a physically relaxing effect and helps towards relaxation. It makes no emotional or dynamic demands on the listener.

My own experience within dance therapy strongly supports the need for careful selection of music, paying attention to such factors as melody, harmony, instrumentation, rhythm and volume. But I would add that the effects are not always common to all, as some music therapists would have us believe. There are significant variables like time, place, group climate, group dynamic, leadership, form and function. Whenever I meet a group for the first time I keep an open mind until I feel able, in some sense to identify the nature of the group. Rarely do I go into a session with specific ideas in a specific order. By the time I am ready to start I have made sure that I am in possession of a fairly good knowledge and understanding as to the nature, conditions and expectations of the group.

Music therapy has a number of applications relevant to dance:

(1) It may overcome self-consciousness over the presence of others.

(2) It may serve as a catalyst in activating unconscious memories or associations.

(3) It may stimulate new moods and impulses.

(4) It can provide a pleasurable sensory kinetic experience.[16]

Drama and dance—drama as therapy

As with music, everything that has so far been said about dance can be said appropriately about drama. Drama constitutes another element in the dance therapy process, providing an additional avenue of consciousness. Through role playing, either real or fictitious, the individual is encouraged to act out his emotional pains and confusions, to project feelings and emotions which have long been repressed. This can be done through a whole drama, role playing with words, or just with movement with music and dance. Gradually the blocked energies and tensions are released, and by bringing the unconscious into the conscious the individual begins to experience release and understand something of his or her dis-ease.

Moreno, one of the founders of pyschodrama, explains:

> When an actor moves out of himself to incorporate the roles and situations in which he has failed, he experiences a 'catharsis of integration'. By acting out the roles of people whom he loves, fears, hates...he learns more about them than he had by actually living with them.

Dance therapy which includes music and drama represents a very rich framework indeed for healing. My own work tends to be with music rather than drama. My concern for drama lies more in a narrative, usually from Scripture or from the individuals' experience, and is used as a means to dance rather than act. I rarely use voice. I have discovered that once the voice is brought in there is an important psychic change from the non-verbal to the verbal. My interest is with expressing in non-verbal terms a basic narrative rather than the narrative itself. The dances included in this publication, and also in *Time to Dance* and *Dance and the Christian Faith,* tend to be concerned with dance and music expressions of a scriptural narrative. The dance and music is designed to express something of the ineffable, heartfelt and spiritual aspect of the narrative in a way that the words cannot.

Notes

1. David Watson, *I Believe in Evangelism* (Hodder and Stoughton: London, 1976).
2. Jane Davies, *The Price of Loving* (Mowbray: Oxford, 1981).
3. Leslie Weatherhead, *Psychology, Religion and Healing.*
4. Thomas Merton, *Conjectures of a Bystander* (Doubleday Image: London, 1968).
5. Susan Langer, *Aesthetic Form and Feeling* (Syracuse, 1958).
6. John Powell, *Why Am I Afraid to Love?* (Fontana: London, 1975).
7. George MacDonald, *Unspoken Sermons.*
8. I Espenak, *Dance Therapy* (C C Thomas).
9. R Arnheim quoted in W Anderson Ed, *Therapy and the Expressive Arts* (Harper and Row: London).
10. Susan Langer, *Feeling and Form* (Routledge and Kegan Paul: London).
11. C S Lewis, *Surprised by Joy* (Fontana: London, 1959).
12. D Eastman, *The Hour that Changed the World* (Baker: Grand Rapids, MI, 1979).
13. Richard Foster, *Celebration of Discipline* (Hodder and Stoughton: London, 1985).
14. *Dance as a Theatre Art* (Dodd and Mead: New York, 1974).
15. J Alvine, *Music Therapy* (Hutchinson: London, 1975).
16. *Ibid.*

6

The Social Dimension of Human Being

Scripture and social health

Social health has as its basis the love of God—the love that causes one to lay down his life for another and that binds the whole together in perfect harmony and unity.

Jesus said: 'A new commandment I give you: Love one another. As I have loved you' (Jn 13:34).

John wrote: 'No-one has ever seen God; but if we love one another, God lives in us and his love is made complete in us' (1 Jn 4:12). 'If anyone says, "I love God," yet hates his brother, he is a liar. For anyone who does not love his brother, whom he has seen, cannot love God, whom he has not seen. . . . Whoever loves God must also love his brother' (1 Jn 4:20, 21).

Reflecting on the nature of the body of Christ, Paul wrote: 'The body is a unit, though it is made up of many parts, and though all its parts are many, they form one body. So it is with Christ' (1 Cor 12:12). 'The eye cannot say to the hand, "I don't need you!" And the head cannot say to the feet, "I don't need you!"' (1 Cor 12:21). 'If one part suffers, every part suffers with it; if one part is honoured, every part rejoices with it' (1 Cor 12:26).

The unity of the body depends upon the love of Christ. Paul urges: 'Get rid of all bitterness, rage and anger, brawling and slander, along with every form of malice. Be kind and compassionate to one another, forgiving each other' (Eph 4:31–32). 'Be completely humble and gentle: be patient, bearing with one another in love. Make every effort to keep the unity of the Spirit through the bond of peace' (Eph 4:2–3).

The power of forgiveness and reconciliation is vital to the health of the community. Jesus said: 'If you are offering your gift at the altar and there remember that your brother has something against you, leave your gift there in front of the altar. First go and be reconciled to your brother' (Mt 5:23–24).

In the same spirit Paul wrote: 'Bear with each other and forgive whatever grievances you may have against one another'. 'Live in harmony with one another,' wrote his fellow Apostle, Peter, 'be compassionate and humble' (1 Pet 3:8).

Writing about forgiveness and healing, James had this to say: 'Is any one of you sick? He should call the elders of the church to pray over him . . . and the prayer offered in faith will make the sick person well; the Lord will raise him up. If he has sinned, he will be forgiven. Therefore confess your sins to each other and pray for each other so that you may be healed' (Jas 5:14–16).

Loving one another in the body of Christ entails mutual respect, sharing and compassion. 'Be devoted to one another in brotherly love. Honour one another above yourselves' (Rom 12:10). 'Share with God's people who are in need' (Rom 12:13). 'Carry each other's burdens, and in this way you will fulfil the law of Christ' (Gal 6:2). 'Encourage the timid, help the weak, be patient with everyone' (1 Thess 5:14).

Living together in loving unity brings with it blessing, as the Psalmist perceived: 'How good and pleasant it is when brothers live together in unity! It is like precious oil poured on the head. . . . It is as if the dew of Hermon were falling on Mount Zion. For there the Lord bestows his blessing, even life for evermore' (Ps 133).

The health of the community

The Christian faith is one that has to be worked out in practical ways, within the context of human relationships. The written word, although primary, can never by itself lead us to faith and growth in God. Until it is made meaningful in action it remains literally a written word. 'There is a tendency more and more,' writes Thomas Merton, 'to preach a "disincarnate word", and to reduce Christ to formal abstract concepts.'[1] The written word, by itself, can never be any more than knowledge 'about' God, 'about' living experience. It cannot ever equal experience. Truth that is not experienced is little better than error. There are some truths which if never experienced never become fully known. The Christian faith is one of those truths.

The truth of the Christian faith, of the love of God, has to be worked out in everyday living and with everyday people. That is true with regard to the mental and physical dimensions of our being, but it is especially true with regard to the social aspect, since the Gospel is essentially a practical, community faith. It is clear that Jesus placed great value on relationships. His teaching is filled with practical suggestions on how to relate to others and maintain relationships. The Sermon on the Mount is particularly relevant with regard to social well-being, but throughout the New Testament generally there is a sustained concern for the importance of healthy relationships.

It is no exaggeration to say that the quality of our human existence is grounded in our relationships. The characteristics frequently identified as constituting a mentally healthy person are summarised by E. M. Layman:

peace of mind
relative freedom from tension and anxiety
feeling of security
sense of self-worth
ability to deal constructively with reality
enjoyment of human contacts
the capacity for mutual satisfaction in social relationships
integration around socially useful values.[2]

What stands out here is the importance of factors that operate on a community level. Layman suggests that, 'considering mental health in a social context, it may be said that mental health is expressed in social health'.

Christianity is a community religion. The Christian is not merely an individual, he belongs as an individual to something larger than himself: he is part of the family of God, the body of Christ. Significantly the numerous instructions in the New Testament epistles are almost exclusively directed towards the church rather than the individual. 'The common word for Christian saint occurs 62 times, 61 in the plural! The overwhelming emphasis is on our corporate life together in Christ. We belong to one another; we are to serve one another.'[3]

'There is no such thing as a solitary Christian! Unless we say, 'Brother', we cannot say, 'Father'! Shutting out our brother shuts out our Father automatically.'[4] Scripture tells us that we cannot love God if we do not love our brothers. Love of God and love of neighbour are not two commandments but one. One learns to love God by loving man. God *is* love and he is found through the love of others. In loving others, and by definition, God, we find our true self. The way of individuation and integration is not a process of detachment, as Thomas Merton recognised: 'Man cannot find himself alone. He must find himself in and through others!'[5] We were created for love, by love, and it is in loving that we find ourselves and our freedom. Only the progress from self-centred love to outgoing love satisfies the divinely placed discontent that exists in each one of us. Ernest Vrisby in his poem 'The Search' writes:

> No one could tell me where my soul might be;
> I sought for God, but God eluded me;
> I sought my brother out and found—all three.[6]

Individual social well-being and community well-being, then, depend upon whether each individual does have a place within the whole, is an indispensable link of the whole. 'Only when even the smallest link is securely interlocked is the chain unbreakable.'[7]

> The physical presence of other Christians should be an incomparable source of joy, and a strength to the believer. There is an infectious happiness in Christians who really love one another, and we should feel no shame about this. It is not a weakness, as though we were still living too much in the flesh, when we yearn for the physical presence of others. Man was created a body, the Son of God appeared on earth in the body. He was raised in the body, in the Sacrament the believer receives the Lord Christ in the body—the believer lauds the Creator, the Redeemer, God, Father, Son and Holy Spirit, for the bodily presence of a brother.[8]

This legitimate loving need we have for each other is not wholly human. While love for another is expressed and experienced through the human body and between human beings, it has its source in something other than, and more than, man. God is love, and the source of the loving need we have for each other is essentially a need to be with God. We are told that while no man has ever seen God, when we love each other God is made real in us through our love for each other. When we love it is not so much 'God is in *my* heart' as 'I am in the heart of God.' That is the nature of Christian love.

It is within the social dimension of our human being particularly that we see love being worked out and made meaningful. And where love is, there is God. Thus the social dimension of being is a great potential source of health and healing.

> When the love of God is in me, God is able to love you, through me, and you are able to love God, through me. If my soul were closed to that love, God's love for you, and your love for God's love for Himself in you and me, would be denied the particular expression which it finds through me, and through no other! Because God's love is in me, it can come to you from a different and special source that could be closed if He did not live in me, and because His love is in you, it can come to me from a quarter from which it would not otherwise come. And because it is in both of us, God has greater glory. His love is expressed in two more ways in which it would not otherwise be expressed: that is, in two more ways that could not exist without Him.[9]

When we give of our personal resources on behalf of someone we care about, a powerful psychic energy is transmitted from within us to the source of our concern, and this seems somehow to activate the natural healing force resident in that person. This subtle healing force, it would appear, stimulates chemical and other agencies in the body that set in action the various psychological processes which are geared to repel infection and reduce the effects of damaging factors in the body's metabolism. The power of love, God's love through each other, represents the most important single source of healing. 'Some day,' wrote Teilhard de Chardin, 'after we have mastered the winds and the waves, the tides and gravity, we will harness for God the energies of love, and then for the second time in the history of the world, man will have discovered fire.'

Deep within each of us is a need to be loved and to love. If

God is love, and we were made *in* love *for* love, the cry of each human being to be loved and to love is essentially that of a creature in relation to its creator. Perhaps this is partly what St Augustine meant when he said: 'Thou madest us for thyself, and our soul is restless till it rest in thee.'

The fact is we cannot do without love—and by definition, without God. A life cut off from love, we are reliably informed by medical research, is a short life. In one study of social isolation it was discovered that the highest incidence of coronary heart disease was found among the most isolated and the lowest among the most social. There are many other consequences, as we shall see later.

> Without love, we lose the will to live. Our mental and physical vitality is impaired, resistance is lowered, and we succumb to illness that often proves fatal. We may escape death, but what remains is a meagre and barren existence, emotionally so impoverished that we can only be called half alive. Life is to be fortified by many friendships. To love and be loved is the greatest happiness of existence. Friendships, above all other relationships, we are discovering, are the springboard to every other love.[10]

Morton Kelsey quotes Bruno Klopfer, the authority of the Rorshach test, as saying:

> 50% of all psychic therapy consists of warm, positive concern. The vast majority of patients whom a physician sees in the course of any given day are there because they do not love themselves or are not loved properly. Many have physical ailments, it is true, but these ailments are essentially physical manifestations of other dis-eases located within the mind, emotions or community.

As another medical writer put it: '90% of all people who come to me would get well if they never saw a physician. They need reassurances, which is another name for love.

Medications, pills, prescriptions, tests and the loving concern that I and my staff give them are symbols of the love they need.' Many doctors willingly admit that pills are often substitutes for the personal time and attention that the doctor cannot give. The more pills a patient receives from the physician, the more they feel he cares for them.

As we saw in the chapter on emotional well-being, we must beware the temptation to refuse either the giving or receiving of love. Thomas Merton reflects:

> Consider the aweful sterility of those who claiming to love God, have in reality dispensed themselves from all obligations to love anyone, and have remained inert and stunted in a little circle of abstract petty concerns involving themselves and a few others as sterile as themselves.

In this increasingly cold, bleak and impersonal world, what people are wanting and needing more than anything else is 'the warmth of love, acceptance and joy. They need to feel God's presence before they will listen to God's word. More than anything, the Church needs to become a loving, caring, welcoming fellowship which radiates the joy of Jesus Christ.'[11] Love, by definition, is social and communal. It can only be realised through another human being.

Wholeness and health are not exclusive to the individual, nor can they be achieved by the individual separate from community. They are a concern for both. The kingdom is not a collection of redeemed individuals, but rather a redeemed community. I am not healthy if I am unhealthily adjusted to community; neither am I healthy if I am well adjusted to an unhealthy community. 'Salvation and wholeness has to do with the social and corporate as well as the individual. It has to do with men in relation to others in community, in the family, home and tribe, in the church and in nations of the world.'[12]

It should be understood that love, which is the essence and central core of our being, while satisfying the deepest needs of our human being, paradoxically, brings with it the deepest and most painful hurts. As one philosopher put it: 'Love is like two porcupines in sub-zero temperatures. In order to survive they need to get close to each other for necessary warmth, but in doing so they prick each other.' Intimacy, which is essential to love, is not all joy. Good friendships are desirable but also dangerous since they are inevitably accompanied by the pains of hurting and being hurt.

To love someone means opening oneself up and making oneself vulnerable. We can only truly love when we are truly ourselves. Love and truth go together. The inevitable consequence of making oneself vulnerable through being open and honest is frequently pain and suffering. Going out to another in love means risk: the risk of self disclosure, rejection and misunderstanding. And the more one becomes involved and open, then the more risk there is of pain and suffering. This is so much so that all too often we close ourselves up and refuse to be 'pricked' any more. This is the paradox of love, and it is precisely within this paradox that the key to truth and to wholeness and health lie. How we resolve, accommodate or reconcile the 'pricks' is essentially what the Christian faith, and health and healing, are all about. It is in the process of resolving these paradoxes that we come to realise and know the Lord, ourselves and each other. How we resolve them will also greatly affect our health and human well-being. And resolve them we must.

Only by withdrawing from our involvement and our loving can we hope to avoid such pain, but this has the effect of producing another sort of pain—a pain arising from loneliness. C S Lewis wrote:

To love at all is to be vulnerable. Love anything, and your heart will certainly be wrung and possibly be broken. If you want to make sure of keeping it intact, you must give your heart to no one, not even to an animal. Wrap it carefully round with hobbies and little luxuries; avoid all entanglements; lock it up safe in the casket or coffin of your selfishness. But in that casket — safe, dark, motionless, airless — it will change. It will not be broken; it will become unbreakable, impenetrable, irredeemable. The alternative to tragedy, or at least to the risk of tragedy, is damnation. The only place outside Heaven where you can be perfectly safe from all the dangers and perturbations of love is Hell. I believe that the most lawless and inordinate loves are less contrary to God's will than a self-invited and self-protective lovelessness . . . we shall draw nearer to God, not by trying to avoid the sufferings inherent in all loves, but by accepting them and offering them to Him; throwing away all defensive armour. [13]

Real love, whatever form it takes, involves commitment. Commitment is essential to love, especially Christian love. Commitment has its roots in faithful obedience to the written word of God as recorded in Scripture. In terms of the Christian community, this means an adherence in faith to the laws of social health and healing as recorded in Scripture. In the same way as God commits himself unconditionally in love to us, so we must each commit ourselves unconditionally to each other. This is the base of Christian commitment.

This commitment, although usually difficult and painful to establish at first, will, as we persevere in faithful obedience to Scripture, begin to grow and develop. And it will grow and develop, paradoxically, out of the pain and failures. The more deeply we commit ourselves to loving relationships, the more we shall hurt. 'As sinners we shall fail and disappoint each other again and again. Yet it is precisely as we accept, with love and understanding, the foibles and frailties of others, the irritating habits that try our patience, the sins that we find we have to forgive, that we shall be fulfilling the law of Christ, the law of love.'[14] 'The development of consciousness is not possible without emotion, and emotion comes to us through the significant relationships in our lives. If we have not loved and hated, been enriched and injured by others, life has not been lived. For this reason relationships are crucial to our psychological development. These relationships must be of the sort that make us vulnerable to being hurt and open to the influence of others.'[15]

One of the real dangers of both psychology and religion is that one may cheat on life. The safe life is not a whole life, and the whole life is not a runaway or pull back to separate oneself from the pain, to erect little barriers, and to protect ourselves from vulnerability. To withdraw or hold back is to destroy, or at least greatly weaken, the love and unity that Christ commanded, prayed for, died for and sent his Spirit to accomplish.

Relationships within many Christian fellowships frequently tend to be superficial and shallow. We may relate to each other in terms of formal worship patterns, and may even greet each other in 'the peace', but for many, fellowship means little more than a casual acquaintance, or at best, a working relationship arising out of the working group which exists for some specific purpose. For most, meetings are little more than conforming interactions between shadows of people rather than honest, intimate human exchanges. Most meetings are based on social habits and external guides, on the values of a system rather than the values of the self or community. 'More often than not, we live in a peace which is not peace, but only escape from an immediate, urgent sense of conflict. It is a peace not of love but anaesthesia. It is a peace not of self-realisation or self-direction but of a flight into irresponsibility.'[16]

Sometimes we are so concerned with the 'ends' of our faith we forget the 'means'. We are so concerned with the super-spiritual that we forget the natural. So concerned with God that misguidedly we forget ourselves and each other. Some-

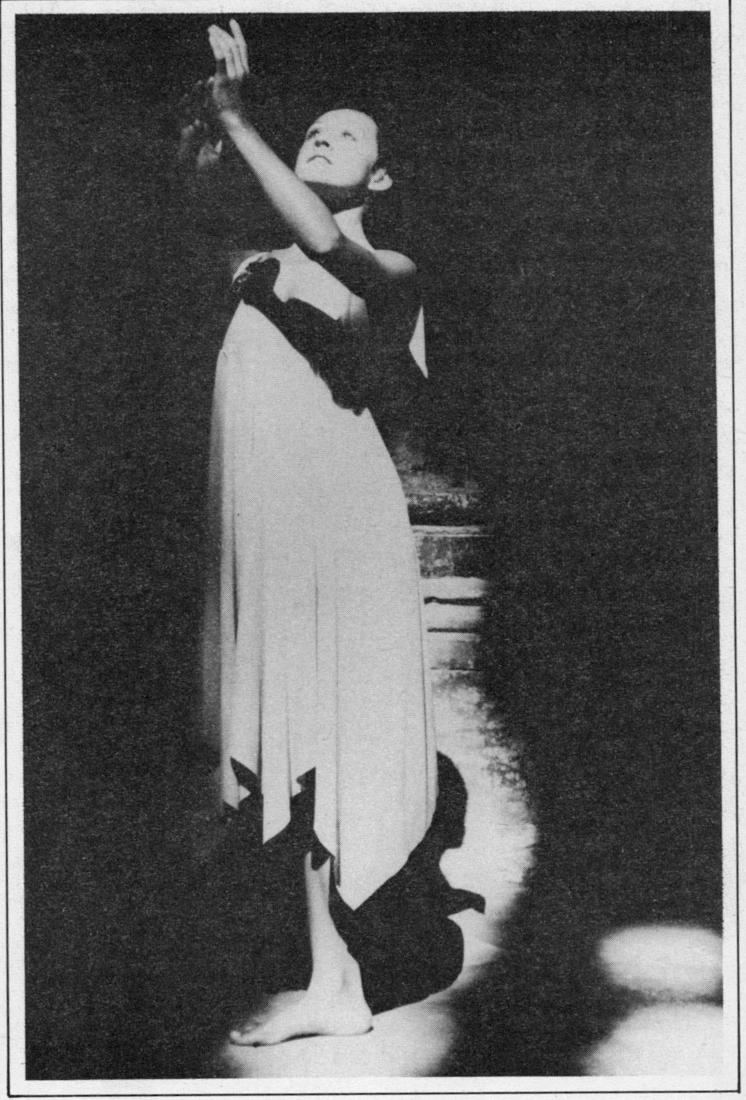

'Create in me a pure heart, O God, and renew a steadfast spirit within me'
(Ps 51:10).

times the church is so concerned with ritual, the mystical, and the life hereafter, that it forgets or seriously undermines the here and now of human being and what that implies.

I am beginning to understand that one of the cruellest and most painful disappointments of my career so far within Christian dance is connected to the paradox of love and the fundamental need for commitment to each other in obedience and faith. During the tour of Western Australia by CDM, at the height of a long and painful process of 'disillusionment', we began, one by one, to withdraw from each other and our ministry. Instead of seeing our hurts, rejections and disappointments as honest expressions of our true selves — our brokenness and helplessness — and as positive points for real growth and development, we eventually allowed our bodies and our worldly thinking to influence our decision to disband. I cannot help wondering what the ministry could have been if we had humbly acknowledged our humanness and somehow managed to fulfil our original commitment to each other and the ministry. 'Only that fellowship which faces disillusionment,' wrote Bonhoeffer, 'with all its unhappy and ugly aspects, begins to be what it should be in God's sight.'

Confrontation in itself does not constitute a positive dynamic within true Christian fellowship, but rather the close and honest sharing and caring that arises out of such confrontations. Moustakis observes:

> I am convinced that it is not confrontation as such but the sharing of one's life with others, the sharing of one's feelings with reference to significant persons in one's world; the sharing of ideas, convictions, values, abilities, feelings, whatever it is that constitutes one's presence as an individual and as a person to a group, the alienating and relational conditions and events. Sharing is the key to intimacy — open, honest, direct, unqualified sharing. I am also convinced that the anguish, the pain, and the suffering that human beings experience and share

with others are more integrative, uniting and connecting emotions in the creation of community life than are the angry encounters and disputes — though it may be necessary to unleash the hostile side before the painful feelings of isolation, loneliness, rejection, terror and inferiority can be expressed and shared.

Confrontation seen positively is a means to deeper intimacy and relatedness, to authenticity between persons. We must be prepared in faith and love to be courageous enough to live through the unknown factors in confrontation, trusting enough to let the breach heal through silent presence and communion when dialogue and words fail, strong enough to maintain a love and respect for each other, whatever else may be cancelled out in the issue or dispute.[17]

The invitation to transparency is not just an invitation to honesty in the recognition of our brokenness and sinfulness; it is also an invitation to 'authenticity'. In ways we do not fully understand, self-disclosure helps us to see things, feel things, imagine things, hope for things, that could never have been possible.

A major find in the subject of self-disclosure is that the human personality has a natural built-in inclination to reveal itself. When that inclination is blocked and we close ourselves to others, we get in emotional trouble. The habitual dissembling and withdrawing leads to disintegration of the personality. Honesty literally can be a health insurance policy, preventing both mental illness and certain kinds of physical sickness . . . we must be prepared to strip ourselves of our masks, make ourselves vulnerable both to God and to each other in order to allow ourselves to be fully known and loved properly as we are.

Following the acknowledgement of our brokenness and sinful state, and our willingness to step out in faith and be authentic in order that we might become whole, is the need for confession and reconciliation. Being our true selves inevitably brings about the need for confession and reconciliation, and in these two activities lies the key to social wholeness and well-being, both individually and collectively.

One of the basic laws of psychology is that until one is accepted and received as one is, no amount of love will bring about the sort of deep and lasting changes necessary for wholeness and well-being. We cannot change anything until we first accept it. Condemnation, either from ourselves or others, does not liberate but oppresses. We should follow the example of our Saviour who, while he in no way condones our sinful behaviour, still accepts us, the sinner. The basis from which we as Christians can speak to one another is that each one of us knows that the other is a sinner, who with all his dignity, is lonely and lost if he is not given help.

Fundamental to community health is the willingness to forgive each other and be reconciled. Many of us find this very difficult to fulfil and find all sorts of excuses for evading it. However logical and convincing in human terms our reasons may seem, they can never, in scriptural terms, constitute reliable and valid excuses. Obedience to the word of Scripture does not rest upon our own logic, especially the logic of a hurt and deceitful heart, but on an obedience, in faith, that God's word is sufficient, just and true. We are called upon to confess to each other and to forgive, whatever the circumstances.

It is with a deep sense of shame I have to admit that within the Christian Dance Ministry there have been times when we have found it very difficult to say sorry and be reconciled. The consequences of disobeying this law have invariably been 'death' — for the individual concerned, the team as a whole and ultimately the ministry. There have been times when I have considered it right to withdraw the team from its engagements until love has been restored. People frequently excuse themselves from reconciliation, and all that this involves, by quoting an old proverb, 'Time will heal.' But time does not in fact heal. It sometimes helps us forget, but that is not the same as healing. Psychology reliably informs us that hurts are repressed or suppressed, held in the unconscious or the subconscious. They continue to affect our behaviour, thoughts and feelings while they remain unresolved. We need to admit that we have done wrong and then ask forgiveness and seek reconciliation. In this way our hurts will be dealt with before they go into the unconscious. This is not just a one-way process. It should be as much the concern of the person receiving the apology as it is of the apologiser (Mt 6:16).

Confessing our sins, hurts and failings to each other in love, as Scripture tells us to do, and reconciling differences, is one of the most powerful of all healing tools. The peace and joy that comes from self-disclosure and being forgiven is an immediate and undeniable release. When we are willing to open up, there is no longer any need to pretend, to repress our weaknesses, to keep up the exhausting effort of playing 'games'. Unconfessed sin keeps us in darkness and breaks our fellowship both with God and each other. He who is alone, as I have personally and painfully learnt, is utterly alone. The more withheld and isolated a person is, the more destructive the power of sin over him, and the more deeply he becomes involved in it. In the darkness of the unexpressed it festers and poisons the whole being, and the fellowship. It tears the body apart. The most expensive thing we can do is to hold the wrong spirit in our hearts against another. When we close our hearts to each other, we close our hearts to God. We are as healthy and whole as we are open and honest with each other.

Why [asks Bonhoeffer] is it often easier to confess our sins to God than to a brother? A brother is sinful as we are. He knows from his *own* experience the dark night of secret sin. Why is it we do not find it easier to go to a brother than to the Holy God? We must ask ourselves whether with our confession of sin to God, we have not rather been confessing our sins to ourselves and granting ourselves absolution. Who can give us the certainty that in the confession and the forgiveness of our sins, we are not dealing with ourselves but with the living God? God gives us the certainty through our *brother*. Our brother breaks the circle of self-deception. A man who confesses his sins in the presence of another knows that he is no longer alone with himself; he experiences the presence of God in the reality of the other person. As long as I am by myself in the confession of my sins everything remains in the dark, but in the presence of a brother the sin has to be brought into the light.[18]

The Christian practice of confession has always been recognised for its therapeutic effect. The Bible commands us: 'Confess your sins to each other . . . so that you may be healed' (Jas 5:16). To persist in ignoring this law of love within the community is to invite the possibility of dis-ease, weakness and even premature death. Bitterness and resentment are frequently a major cause of unhappiness in Christian fellowships. They breed depression and disease, and freeze the river of joy in a Christian's soul. Such may seem rather exaggerated by some, but current medical findings show that such negative relationships and highly charged feelings sustained over a period of time can and do drastically alter the body's metabolism to produce harmful effects.

For centuries scoffers have ridiculed the advice of Jesus to 'love one's enemies'. They scorned it as impractical, idealistic, and absurd. Now psychiatrists have shown that this radical and life changing attitude would prevent many of the ills man brings upon himself through resentment of his enemies.[19]

It takes considerable strength and maturity to own up and take on the responsibility for one's sin. It takes even more strength and maturity to take on the responsibility for the sin of another brother or sister who is unable or unwilling to recognise his or her part in the sin. Whatever our part in the dis-eased relationship, each person has a responsibility to forgive and reconcile. A submission is certainly involved, but it is rooted in love, not weakness. Nothing contributes more to sickness than resentment and bitterness, and nothing contributes more to health and healing than to forgive and forget.

In recent years there has been a significant development in social 'medicine', especially small group therapy. In socio and psychodrama, dance and music therapy, group dynamics, self-help groups, sensitivity groups, personal growth groups, etc, we see various attempts to meet some of the needs of social and psychological dis-ease, maladjustment and deprivation arising from an isolated, fragmented and alienating society. A brief look at some of the reasons for this development will help us understand some of the major concerns of social health and healing.

Rolo May considers that it reflects the disintegration of our culture and, more particularly, the social bonds that bind us together and support us through difficult periods in our lives. 'Never', she writes, 'has relationship appeared as complex and difficult as it appears today, and never has the search for valued relationships and a community been more urgent and intense. More and more people are turning to psychiatry and psychotherapy for help in this search.[20]

Carl Rogers, another pioneer in psychotherapy, and originally a theological student, sees it as a significant part of the attempt to meet the isolation of contemporary life. He writes:

> We are sufficiently affluent that our physical needs are met, and now, what would we most like to have? We would like to be free from the alienation that is so much a part of urban life, and so much a part of life in general. We would like, somehow, to find ourselves in real contact with other persons. I believe this desire is one of the elements that gives much of the magnetism to the intensive group experience.

Frank Hardy, in *The Unlucky Country: A picture of Australia*, writes:

> We didn't talk much. If he spoke at all it was about trucks, traffic, policemen, transport officials, truck drivers, unhitching unwilling women hitch-hikers. Once he bemoaned being back on the long haul after eighteen months driving round Sydney. He didn't know who I was, didn't ask any questions. And I resisted the lifelong habit of a geniality that holds back the essential self, the ready friendliness that makes it easy to know a man a little and impossible to know him well — the Australian gregariousness that leads a man to a loneliness where he knows everyone yet no one.

We have, it seems, begun to recognise the limit of what material things can give the individual in the way of fulfilment. We are now turning to the psychological world in an attempt to find something that will give satisfaction, something that will permit a more profound and authentic realisation of one's human being. 'I believe this whole development has a special significance for a culture which appears bent on dehumanising the individual and dehumanising our interpersonal relations. The phenomenon of the group enterprise is an important force in the opposite direction, a direction toward making relationships more meaningful and more personal.'[21]

But perhaps the most significant observation about social health comes from Carl Rogers once again:

> Psychotherapy is meeting needs formerly met by organised religion; many of the new (and secular) therapies have profoundly religious overtones. So do many of the more orthodox forms of counselling, which derive much of their energy from spiritual notions of rebirth and growth, redemption and salvation, the healing power of love and the essential goodness of man. These ideas are couched in secular and psychological terms, so that

often their religious nature remains concealed, but they nevertheless, remain essentially religiously based.

How does the church fit into all this we may well ask? How is
it that the secular social sciences have taken from the church
that which was originally its proper concern? The heart of the
Gospel is fundamentally social. Why is it that the socially
dis-eased no longer come to the church for help? Is the church
so irrelevent, so exclusive, so uncompassionate? F Rokeach
reveals from a study of religious people in USA—irrespective
of whether religion was defined in terms of nominal identification, church attendance, or its self-rated salience—that
they were in fact socially *less* compassionate that the non-
religious. The religious placed more emphasis on personal
salvation and were more anxious to maintain the status quo,
they were more unsympathetic to blacks, the poor, and
student protest movement that the non-religious. Rokeach
suggests a portrait of the religious-minded church-goer as
'one who has a self-centred pre-occupation with the saving of
his own soul, and an alienated, otherwordly-orientation
coupled with indifference toward—and tacit endorsement
of—a social system that would perpetuate social inequality
and injustice. Moreover, the results seem compatible with
the hypothesis that religious values serve more as standards
for condemning others, or as standards to rationalise one's
own self pursuit than standards to judge one's own self by or
to guide one's own conduct.[22]

The validity and reliability of this piece of research is not as
important as the questions it raises. There is some truth, it
has to be admitted, in what is being said. But the important
thing for us is, how we as a church fellowship can alleviate
such social pain and suffering. Perhaps we could start with
ourselves as a social body, but not for exclusively selfish
reasons. It seems to me that there is as much loneliness and
social dis-ease within the church fellowship as there is
without. David Watson writes:

Our Churches are filled with people who, outwardly, look contented and at peace, but inwardly, are crying out for someone to love them—confused, frustrated, often frightened, and guilty, they are often unable to communicate even within their own formulas. When other people look so happy and contented in the Church, one seldom has the courage to admit one's own deep needs before such self sufficiency, as the average church meeting appears to be.[23]

Helping, encouraging and supporting each other, listening to and expressing care for each other, is not the exclusive task of the professional counsellor. It is the commission of every Christian (Gal 6:2; Phil 2:4). Religion is not something separate from everyday life and everyday people. It is, or should be, concerned with everyday life and everyday people. All too often I have found in my experience that the church, and I include myself, like Malvolio in Shakespeare's *Twelfth Night,* is more in love with the idea of being in love, than love itself. For many, the Christian faith is a substitution, frequently a romantic and idealistic one, for real life.

The church [writes Jerome Liss] should be a laboratory of love where a person experiences the giving and receiving of acceptance, forgiveness, understanding and concern. It should be a listening and supporting group where persons grow to listen with an openness and positive interest, with a sacrificial involvement: with expectancy so great as to evoke the fullest capacities from each other, with patience grounded in faith in what the person may become: without judgement but with deep concern.[24]

I propose now to look, in general terms, at some of the research findings arising out of this growing concern for social dis-ease and small group therapy, and see if there is anything that might encourage us as a Christian community to consider more carefully and more realistically some of the laws of Scripture as they affect social health and healing.

First, what do people who attend these group therapies

expect from such an experience? One piece of research reveals that the large majority — more than 70% of 500 persons — indicated the following:

Rank	Expectation	%
1	Increased capacity for developing relationships	88
2	Finding out how others really see me	88
3	Being able to express my feelings	87
4	Being sensitive to other's feelings	86
5	Being able to share things with others and get close	84
6	Experiencing joy and self-fulfilment	83
7	Changing some of the ways I relate to people	80
8	Meeting new people and making friends	78
9	Being able to help and support others	76
10	Understanding my inner self	76
11	Having new experiences	70[25]

Subsequent research would strongly support the view that people who engage in such group processes do, in fact, experience such significant changes in their behaviour as a direct result of the small group experience. Among such beneficial effects are:

increase in self-esteem
self-concept changes in many positive directions
alienation is reduced
individual problems are lessened
interpersonal relationships become more emphatic and improved
people become closer and feel less lonely

J R Gibbs reinforces these findings:

more sensitive towards social reality — increased awareness
self-actualisation
authentic experience — increase in validity and reliability of
    behaviour which emphasises openness and authenticity, con-
    gruence, transparency and confrontation.
creative release experiences
a reduction of fears and inhibitions
increased spontaneity
practical expression of coping behaviour
increased communication

Perhaps one of the most comprehensive pieces of recent research is that by Argyle and Henderson.[26] Based on extensive findings of recent research, it sets out to explore the structure of different types of relationships, examining their essential features, the formal and informal rules.

Argyle and Henderson support the notion that 'satisfactory relationships benefit the whole person — mental, emotional, physical and social' and that unsatisfactory relationships lead to mental, physical, emotional and social dis-ease. Gaining a relationship represents 'one of the pleasantest and most posi-tive life events', while losing one represents 'the worst and most distressing'. Making a new friend was rated more positive than winning a lot of money, job promotion, a pay rise, going on holiday, buying a new home or a new car! Those who are married, who have lots of friends, or who in other ways have a supportive network, are happier, in better physical and mental health, and live longer. Research into loneliness shows that people who feel lonely, also feel unhappy, depressed, worthless, anxious, lacking self-esteem, bored and so on. Among adolescents and students, loneliness was found to be particularly widespread. In a survey of over 100,000 American men and women it was found that 'being in love' was rated second to 'friends and social life' for single men and women.

Rules of friendship were found to include:

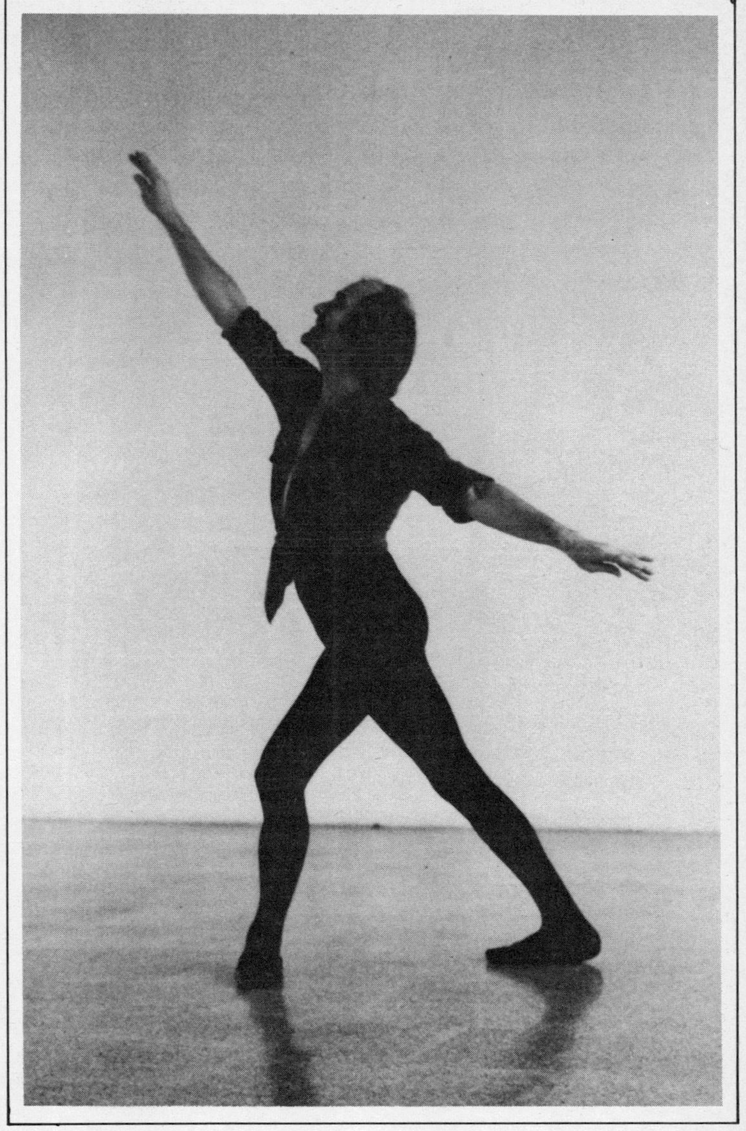

'Those who hope in the Lord will renew their strength' (Is 40:31).

volunteer help in time of need
respect the friend's privacy
keep confidences
trust and confide in each other
stand up for a friend
do not criticise in public
share emotional support
look in the eye in conversation
strive to make each other happy
do not be jealous or critical of other relationships
toleration of one's friends
share news of success
ask personal advice
don't nag
seek to repay debts and favours
compliment each other
disclose personal feelings and problems

Contact with friends seems to be important for the young and old; it may be less so in between. What is important is not the *quantity* of social interaction as the *quality*. This includes such behaviour as:

the level of intimacy — this is a particularly important element
    in friendship and the eradication of loneliness
the amount of self-disclosure
the pleasantness of contact
the satisfaction derived from it

Relationships help by providing:

intimate close attachments of caring, trust and empathy
confidantes — psychotherapeutic
affirmation — giving confidence, self-esteem and an
    ability to cope
tangible help
information help
social integration

We express and reflect intimacy by:

addressing the other person by first name
showing an interest in the other person's activity
sharing news of success
trusting and confiding
sharing other person's position unconditionally
acknowledging birthdays and special occasions
striving to make the other happy while in his company
inviting him to family celebrations or other intimate affairs
making the other welcome
showing affection
discussing intimate topics

There is much evidence to suggest that stress makes people ill by undermining the immune system, the body's natural defence against germs. It seems likely that by reducing social stress, social support can greatly assist to keep the immune system operating. Another possibility is that the relaxation response is actuated by social support: this in turn reverses the biochemical effects of stress.[27]

Like many Christians involved with health and healing, the more I become acquainted with the principles of holistic health, the more I realise that the church holds one of the major keys to human well-being in that it can, or should, be a loving community. The early Christians were known for precisely this. Selwyn Hughes writes:

The Church of Christ, when functioning in harmony with God's principles, can do as much, if not more, to bring wholeness as the skills of doctors. The majority of people who are experiencing physical problems can be tremendously helped by the warm, genuine, interest of people who care.[28]

The church of tomorrow which moves with power and proclaims with any authority the kingdom of God, will have to be familiar with the findings of depth psychology and use these findings to minister not only to the wounded and broken of the world, but to its own people.[29]

All too often in my experience of the church, especially theological colleges, concern is almost exclusively theological and historical with little regard for the disciplines of psychology and sociology as they relate to real life. In contemporary research from psychology and sociology we see what was revealed by God to man many hundreds of years ago. Books such as *Anatomy of Relationships* and *None of these Diseases* are essentially rediscoveries of ancient truths.

On a final and perhaps controversial note, given the present arguments about the place of women in the church, Argyle and Henderson's research reveals that 'women form much more intimate and effective friendships than men, and that they are a better cure for loneliness in others than are male friendships.' The research actually goes on to reveal much about the nature and conditions of such differences between men and women, which I believe are important to the church.

I emphasised at the beginning of my writing that the focus of this book is not on dance for its own sake, but rather as a means to health and healing. Perhaps this is no more strongly expressed than in this fourth dimension of human being. I have given considerable space and attention to Scripture and social psychology rather than dance because it is necessary to understand something about the nature and conditions of social health before one can understand how dance can help.

Health and healing is a large ministry demanding a wide variety of gifts and disciplines which can, through the richness of God's grace, bring true healing to the total brokenness of man. Dance, one of man's most primary forms of expression represents one of these many and diverse avenues through which human wholeness and well-being may be attained and retained.

Dance

The Christian dance group is essentially a fellowship made up of Christians. As part of the wider church it is a place where each can live and work out his or her faith according to Scripture. This entails using dance to bring social health and healing according to Scripture.

As we have already observed, there is a remarkable similarity between Scripture and contemporary psychotherapy in their basic assumptions about man, the ends of man, and the means whereby such ends should be realised. All the benefits for health and healing claimed by psychotherapy, and substantiated by scientific research, may be applied to Christian health and healing, and dance therapy especially. Dance therapists claim such benefits as:

an increased capacity for interaction and developing relationships
finding out how others see us—strengthening identity concept
learning how to contain and release feelings in socially acceptable
   terms
being able to express feelings
being sensitive to others
being able to share with others and develop a social intimacy
being able to make new friends
experience joy and fulfilment: emotional, physical and social

This, of course is hardly new, as we discussed very early on in this book. Dance has always been a means towards social, emotional and physical health and healing—even at the level of everyday community life. It remains so today, implicitly at least, in much recreation and dance. In the 1960s Frances Rust identified some of the values adolescents in colleges and polytechnics placed on ballroom and jive dance:

everyone can enjoy themselves and be relaxed
it helps the atmosphere and therefore one enjoys the occasion
    better
it's relaxing, provides a good social evening
good energetic expression
a means of self-expression
allows you to express your feelings
it's not so much the dance I like — it's the atmosphere
the music and the chance it provides for meeting other people
sensational, intimate and sexy
allows a formal contact with another person
you can really dance with all you are and have fun
good way of getting rid of natural exuberance
graceful, sophisticated, beautiful
outlet for energy
a means of escape
express feelings more easily
an opportunity to express freely without self-consciousness or
    being ridiculed socially
useful socially
mentally relaxing
induces a spirit of enjoyment, happiness
everyone can have a go — everyone can join in, it's for all

It should be noted that among the above reasons for dancing the emphasis is not exclusively social. The physical, emotional and mental are equally important justifications in the eyes of these young people. Among the many social benefits claimed for dance therapy are:

participation is the first step in socialisation; through expressive
    movement in the group, the individual learns to share feelings
    with others and recognise that he is not alone
participation affords channels for making social contacts within
    a secure, formal and socially acceptable setting
participation creates a feeling of security and oneness for the
    socially/emotionally withdrawn; merely holding the hands of

another and facing another can represent a healthy step forward

participation helps break down barriers of isolation and dependency

contributes to a growing sense of group consciousness

provides a friendly, supportive, encouraging and accepting atmosphere within which the dis-eased member may begin to grow and develop

for the awkward and self-conscious—social participation is possible

become more and more at ease, more comfortable within the dance therapy group

social/emotional contact is usually easier to establish in non-verbal dance—both with oneself and others

simple folk dance provides maximum participation with the minimum amount of frustration by building up the individual's confidence of being able to work within the group

in the dance therapy group the member experiences acceptance and approval in participation with others which is both pleasurable and gratifying

a channel for uninhibited drives into socially acceptable expressions

builds up social solidarity

helps one relate to others one can trust

shyness, withdrawal and hostility are gradually reduced

protective social/emotional barriers begin to come down

a feeling of openness and trust through physical and social encounter quickly develop

for those insecure in their social contacts, such participation with others in the dance, in a non-threatening situation, can help build up the self-esteem and self-reliance so necessary for social adjustment

in group dancing the emphasis is on doing things together; this tends to produce feelings of empathy among participants

the situation is set up variously as permissive, admiring, praising, accepting, safe, gratifying, reassuring, supporting, non-threatening, non-comparing and non-judgemental

Notice how these claims overlap and reinforce each other; and notice also that while 'these justifications may not belong to art, and may not be included in investigations led by aestheticians they nevertheless constitute an essential part of human development'.[30]

Finally, an extract from Cecil Sharpe, a devoted pioneer of dance of the community — folk dance:

> Folk dance was not concerned with ceremonial and formality. It was, and so far as it is practised, still is the ordinary everyday dance of the country folk, performed not merely on feast days, but whenever opportunity offered and the spirit of merrymaking was abroad. It was performed in groups, in couples, or with partners of the opposite sex. No special dress was needed. The steps and figures were easily learned . . . it was always danced for its own sake, for the pleasure it afforded the 'performer' and the social intercourse that it provided.[31]

In dance as social therapy, priority is given to the inter-personal relationships within the group, to the climate of love, encouragement and support. It is the dance therapist's effectiveness in establishing such an environment which encourages the dis-eased participants to open themselves up, both to themselves and to each other, in order that they can begin to be authentic and grow.

Notes

1. Thomas Merton, *Conjectures of a Bystander* (Doubleday Image: London, 1968).
2. E M Layman, *Science and Medicine of Exercise and Sports* (Harper and Row: London).
3. David Watson, *Discipleship* (Hodder and Stoughton: London, 1983).
4. Selwyn Hughes, *Everyday with Jesus Daily Notes*.
5. Thomas Merton, *No Man Is an Island* (Burns and Oates:

Tunbridge Wells, 1974).
6. Ernest Vrisby quoted in A L Allen, *God's Psychiatry* (Power Books: Old Tappan, NJ).
7. Dietrich Bonhoeffer, *Life Together* (SCM: London, 1954).
8. *Ibid.*
9. Thomas Merton, *New Seeds of Contemplation* (New Directions, 1961).
10. Alan McGinnis, *The Friendship Factor* (Hodder and Stoughton: London, 1983).
11. David Watson, *I Believe in Evangelism* (Hodder and Stoughton: London, 1976).
12. John Baker, *Salvation and Wholeness* (Fountain Trust, 1973).
13. C S Lewis, *The Four Loves* (Fontana: London, 1963).
14. David Watson, *Discipleship*.
15. J A Sandford, *Healing and Wholeness* (Paulist Press).
16. Thomas Merton, *op cit*.
17. Clarke Moustakas, *Individuality and Encounter* (Howard and Doyle, 1968).
18. Dietrich Bonhoeffer, *op cit*.
19. H C Link *None of these Diseases* (Lakeland: Basingstoke).
20. Rolo May, 'Psychotherapy and the Search for Meaning'. *The Listener* (November, 1978).
21. N Solomon, *New Perspectives on Encounter Groups* (Jossey Bass: London, 1972).
22. F Rokeach, 'Faith, Hope and Bigotry', *Psychology Today* vol 3 no 58 (1970).
23. David Watson, *op cit*.
24. Jerome Liss, *Free to Feel* (Wildwood House).
25. J Bebout and B Gordin quoted in *New Perspectives on Encounter Groups*.
26. Argyle and Henderson, *Anatomy of Relationships* (Penguin: London, 1985).
27. W E Broadbent, 'The Epidemiological Evidence for Relationship between Social Support and Health', *Journal of Epidemiology* vol 117 (1983).
28. Selwyn Hughes, *God Wants You Whole* (Kingsway: Eastbourne, 1984).
29. Elizabeth O'Connor, *Journey Inward, Journey Outward* (Harper

and Row: London, 1968).

30. R Laing, *The Nature of Dance* (MacDonald and Evans: Plymouth).

31. Cecil Sharpe, *The Country Dance Book* (EP: London, 1972).

PART 3

Practical Dance

Song numbers in this section refer to the Integrated Music and Words editions of *Songs and Hymns of Fellowship* (designated here as *SoF*) published by Kingsway. All music and words are reproduced by permission of the copyright holders.

1. *Be Still and Know*

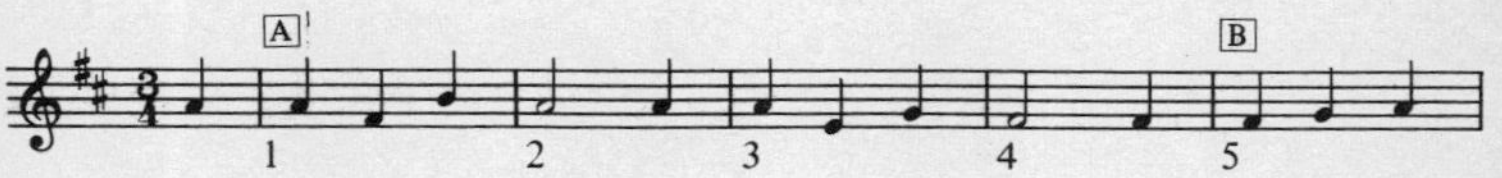

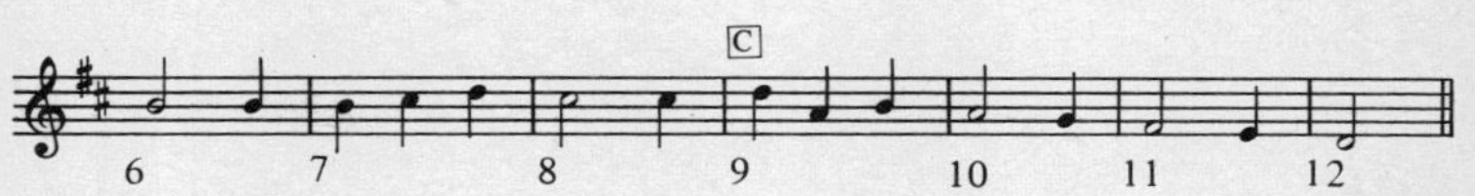

Be still and know that I am God,
Be still and know that I am God,
Be still and know that I am God.

Author unknown. *SoF 37*

MUSIC	BAR	BEAT	MOVEMENT
'placing'			**Starting position** Each dancer, identified as 'a', 'b' or 'c' and carefully placed as such, sits back on the R/l, with the L/f firmly planted on the ground ready to take the body weight onto it in order to rise on that L/l. The position is one of quiet supplication, with the arms held loosely and slightly away from the body, palms open and forward, the head tilted forward.
A	1–4		**Verse one** During the first four bars, remain still.
B			The group identified as 'a', 'b' and 'c' one at a time, in canon, slowly bring their heads up to gaze at the cross. At the same time arms move a little further away from the side. The chest is lifted.
	5		Group 'a' slowly bring their heads up.
	6		Group 'b' slowly bring their heads up.
	7		Group 'c' slowly bring their heads up.
	8		All hold – still.
C	9–12		Leading with the chest, and the face focused high upon the cross, all slowly rise by bringing the weight onto the L/l. Quietly and confidently, come to stand tall. Keep the arms held loosely away from the sides with the palms open and forward.

MUSIC	BAR	BEAT	MOVEMENT
A	1–4		**Verse two** 'Be still…'
B			The group identified as 'a', 'b' and 'c' slowly, in three-part canon, bring their arms out forwards/diagonally to high and wide above the head with palms open and horizontal, the arms slightly contracted.
	5		Group 'a' slowly bring their arms up.
	6		Group 'b' slowly bring their arms up.
	7		Group 'c' slowly bring their arms up.
	8		Hold – still.
C	9–12		The group lower their arms in unison and return them to their position of being held loosely at the side. The face remains focused high upon the cross.
A	1–4		**Verse three** 'Be still…'
			The group identified as 'a', 'b', and 'c' slowly sink to their original position by taking the R/l back, coming to sit back on it. This is done, once again, in three-part canon.

MUSIC	BAR	BEAT	MOVEMENT
B	5		Group 'a' slowly sink.
	6		Group 'b' slowly sink.
	7		Group 'c' slowly sink.
	8		Hold – still.
C	9–10		All slowly tilt the head forward.
	11–12		All slowly bring the head forward and high once again to the cross. At the same time, bring the arms diagonally forward at the waist level, with the palms open and upturned…in quiet supplication.

'Be still and know that I am God…I am the Lord that healeth…put your trust in me.'

Stillness…in this movement expression is a metaphor related to the whole of one's being—mental, emotional, physical, spiritual and social—rather than simply physical.

Remember that 'stillness'—and all that is implied by such a concept—does not lie in the movement instructions themselves. The movement suggestions are but vehicles which you, the dancer, are invited to bring alive by investing something of yourself in them.

As you meditate on the words and meanings with your mind, heart, body, and together as a fellowship, let each aspect of your being affect the other until the whole is saturated with the meaning and purpose of this Scripture. Let something of this experience be expressed in the dance.

An alternative 'developed' idea

Using the same material of the established three verses, the whole can be performed as a three-part canon. Each of the three groups 'a', 'b' and 'c' simply begins with a different verse. For example:

> Group 'a' begins with the material of verse one—kneeling.
> Group 'b' begins with the material of verse two—standing.
> Group 'c' begins with the material of verse three—standing.

2. *In Thy Presence*

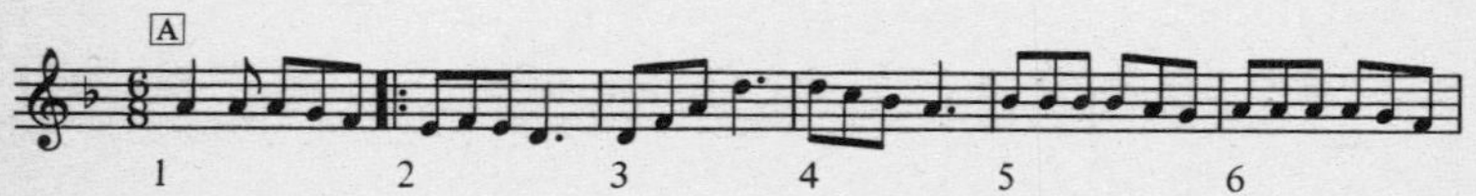

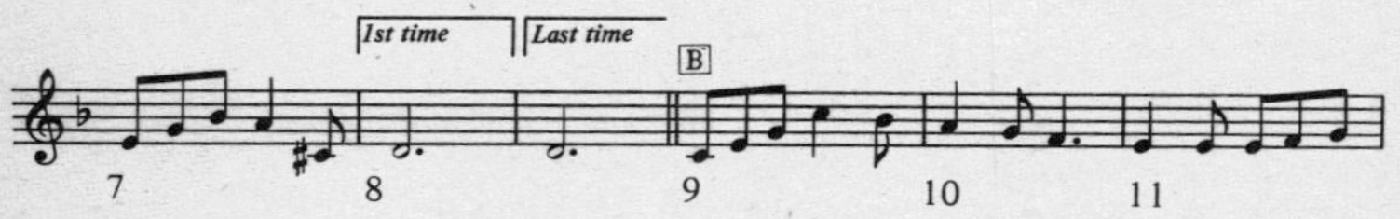

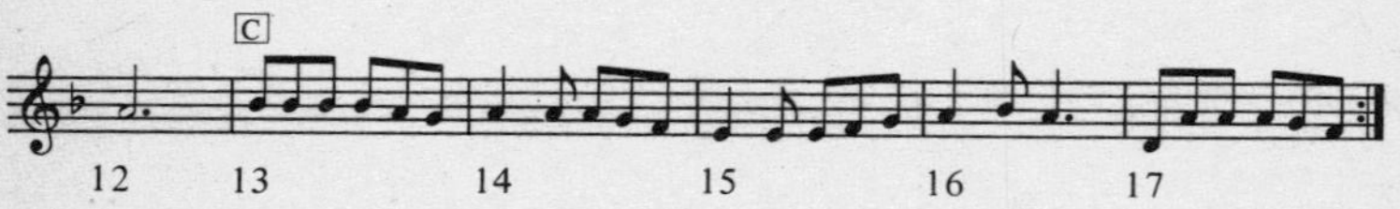

In Thy presence there's fullness of joy,
Fullness of joy, fullness of joy.
At Thy right hand are pleasures for ever,
Pleasures for evermore.

I keep the Lord before me,
I shall not be moved.
My heart is glad and my soul rejoices,
I shall dwell in safety.

Mike Kerry. © 1982 Thankyou Music, P.O. Box 75, Eastbourne BN23 6NW. *SoF 223*

MUSIC	BAR	BEAT	MOVEMENT
			Starting position The dancers, identified as 'a' and 'b' alternately and as partners, form a circle facing the centre with hands held at shoulder level ready to side skip to the left.
A	1	1 3 4 6	**Chorus** Step L/f to L Close R/f to L/f Step L/f to L Close R/f to L/f } skip sideways to the left
	2	1 3 4 6	Step L/f to L Close R/f to L/f Step L/f to L Hop L/f
	3	1 3 4 6	Step R/f forward Hop R/f Step L/f forward Hop L/f } skip forwards into the centre, or walk if preferred
	4	1 3 4 6	Step R/f backward Hop R/f Step L/f backward Hop L/f } skip backwards out of the centre, or walk if preferred
	5	1 3 4 6	Step R/f to R Close L/f to R/f Step R/f to R Hop R/f } skip to right

MUSIC	BAR	BEAT	MOVEMENT
	6	1	Step L/f to L
		3	Close R/f to L/f
		4	Step L/f to L
		6	Hop L/f } skip to left
	7	1	Step R/f to R
		3	Close L/f to R/f
		4	Step R/f to R
		6	Close L/f to R/f } pivot turn to
	8	1	Step R/f to R the R on the R/f.
		3	Close L/f to R/f
		4	Step R/f to R
		6	Hop R/f
B	9	1	**Variation B1** Step L/f forward
		4	Step R/f forward } walk into the circle
	10	1	Step L/f forward
		4	Step R/f forward
	11	1	Step L/f back
		3	Hop L/f
		4	Step R/f back
		6	Hop R/f } skip out of the circle
	12	1	Step L/f back
		3	Hop L/f
		4	Step R/f back
		6	Hop R/f

MUSIC	BAR	BEAT	MOVEMENT
C	13–16		At this point 'a's turn to their left and 'b's turn to their right, all perform the folk dance motif, 'the hey', for the next four bars finishing facing, the centre of the circle, ready to pick up the Chorus once again, ie each person walks the way he is facing, and greets a new partner every two steps by shaking hands, first with the R/hand then the L, and so on.
			Repeat Chorus, ie go back to the beginning. On the completion of the Chorus for the second time move to variation B2.
B	9	1 4	**Variation B2** 'a's turn to their left and 'b's to their right. Perform the folk motif 'step-and-turn'. Step L/f to L Place R/f next to L—keep body weight on L/f.
	10	1 4	Step R/f to R Place L/f next to R—keep body weight on R/f.
	11	1 4	Step L/f Step R/f } individual circle to the
	12	1 4	Step L/f } left on the spot. Step R/f
C	13–16		Arming — Link R arm with the R arm of your partner and either walk or skip around for two bars, finishing ready to go back to the Chorus once again. Finish at the end of Chorus.

MUSIC	BAR	BEAT	MOVEMENT
	17		Repeat Chorus and finish.

The structure of this dance is a 'rondo':

Chorus
Variation   B1
Chorus
Variation   B2
Chorus

There is no reason why you could not add another variation
or perhaps continue the music and encourage the
congregation to join you in a simple farandole idea where
one of the dancers simply leads a chain with everyone
joining hands and following the leader.

3. *O Let the Son of God Enfold You*

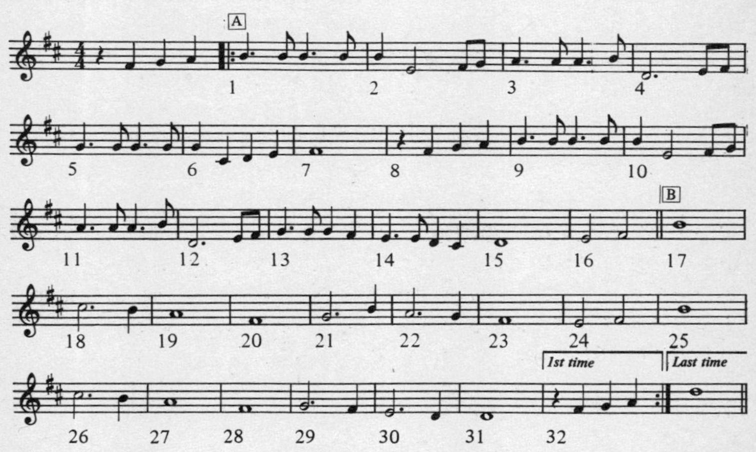

O let the Son of God enfold you
With His Spirit and His love,
Let Him fill your heart and satisfy your
  soul.
O let Him have the things that hold you,
And His Spirit like a dove
Will descend upon your life and make
  you whole.

Jesus, O Jesus,
Come and fill your lambs.
Jesus, O Jesus,
Come and fill Your lambs.

O come and sing this song with gladness
As your hearts are filled with joy,
Lift your hands in sweet surrender to
  His name.
O give Him all your tears and sadness,
Give Him all your years of pain,
And you'll enter into life in Jesus'
  name.

MUSIC	BAR	BEAT	MOVEMENT
	$+$ a b c d		**Starting position** Dancers, identified as 'a', 'b', 'c' and 'd', kneel on R/knee, head is tilted forward and arms are held loosely out to the side. The posture is one of quiet submission.
A	1–2		'O let the Son of God enfold you' Slowly the head comes up to gaze up at the cross. At the same time the arms come slightly forward and out to the side with palms upturned.
	2–4		'With His Spirit and His love' Slowly lower the head once again and bring the arms across one's chest, wrists crossing and hands open. Remain very relaxed. Keep the arms slightly away from the body.
	4–8		'Let Him fill your heart and satisfy your soul' Keeping the head lowered, at first, and the wrists crossed, bring the arms up and over the head, then release the whole and bring the arms high and wide above the head, with palms upturned and horizontal. Slowly bring them down to the original position. At the same time lower the head ready to repeat the whole sequence.
	9–16		Repeat bars 1–8 'O let Him have the things that hold you, and His Spirit like a dove will descend upon your life and make you whole'

MUSIC	BAR	BEAT	MOVEMENT
			Each group in turn, at a one bar interval slowly bring the arms outwards diagonally forwards and up to high and wide above the head, at the same time letting the weight of the body come forwards onto the supporting leg and lifting the whole torso. The effect is a combination of reaching out and lifting up, petitioning and praise.
B	17		Group 'a'—slowly begin to bring arms up.
	18		Group 'b'—slowly begin to bring arms up.
	19		Group 'c'—slowly begin to bring arms up.
	20		Group 'd'—slowly begin to bring arms up. NB Each group must take four bars to complete the arm sequence. The effect is a four-part canon, each group following the other. This is carried over for the next 12 bars.
	21		Group 'a'—slowly begin to bring arms down.
	22		Group 'b'—slowly begin to bring arms down.
	23		Group 'c'—slowly begin to bring arms down.
	24		Group 'd'—slowly begin to bring arms down.

MUSIC	BAR	BEAT	MOVEMENT
	25—32		Repeat bars 17—24.
			All should finish together in bar 32 ready to go back to the beginning.

4. *Jubilate Deo*

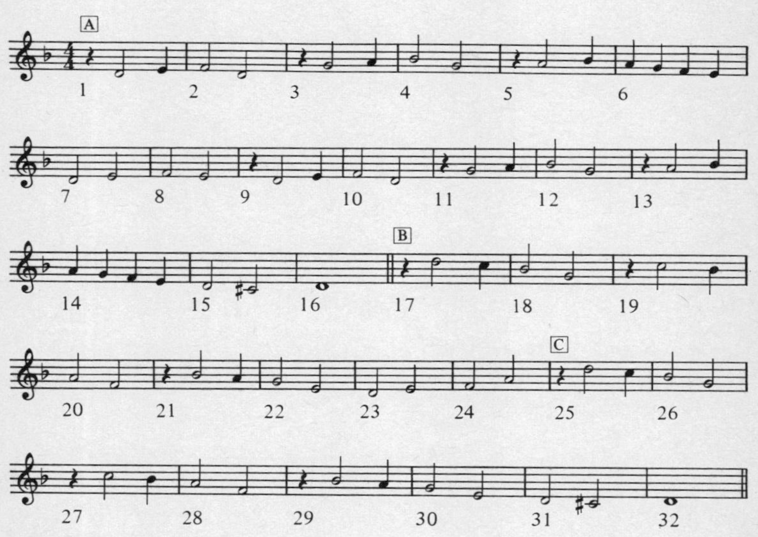

Jubilate, everybody,
Serve the Lord in all your ways
And come before His presence singing,
Enter now His courts with praise.
For the Lord our God is gracious,
And His mercy everlasting.
Jubilate, Jubilate, Jubilate Deo.

Fred Dunn. © 1977, 1980 Thankyou Music, P. O. Box 75, Eastbourne BN23 6NW. *SoF 303*

MUSIC	BAR	BEAT	MOVEMENT
			Starting position Dancers, identified as 'a' and 'b' alternately, stand facing the centre of the circle, hands held at shoulder level, ready to move off and face left.
A	1	1 3	Step R/f across L/f Step L/f side L
	2	1 3	Step R/f behind L/f Step L/f side L
	3	1 3	Step R/f across L/f Step L/f side L
	4	1 3	Step R/f behind Step L/f side travel left.
	5	1 3	Step R/f across L/f Step L/f side L
	6	1 3	Step R/f behind Step L/f side
	7	1 3	Step R/f across L/f Step L/f *back* behind R 'mark time'.
	8	1 3	Step R/f across L/f Hop R/f

MUSIC	BAR	BEAT	MOVEMENT	
	9	1	Step L/f behind R/f	
		3	Step R/f side	
	10	1	Step L/f across R/f	
		3	Step R/f side	travel right.
	11	1	Step L/f behind R/f	
		3	Step R/f side R	
	12	1	Step L/f across R/f	
		3	Hop L/f	
	13	1	Step R/f back	release hands to
		3	Step L/f forward	perform an
	14	1	Step R/f forward	individual half-
		3	Step L/f forward	circle on the spot, to the left.
	15—16		'Pivot turn', R/f to the R, ending with a hop on the R/f ready for the next motif.	

MUSIC	BAR	BEAT	a	b
B	17	1	Step L/f forward	Step L/f backward
		2	Hop L/f	Hop L/f
		3	Step R/f forward	Step R/f backward
		4	Hop R/f	Hop R/f
	18	1	Step L/f forward	Step L/f backward
		2	Hop L/f	Hop L/f
		3	Step R/f forward	Step R/f backward
		4	Hop R/f	Hop R/f
			Arms come across the body and up, high and wide above the body in an expression of jubilation.	

MUSIC	BAR	BEAT	MOVEMENT	
	19	1 2 3 4	Step L/f backward Hop L/f Step R/f backward Hop R/f	Step L/f forward Hop L/f Step R/f forward Hop R/f
	20	1 2 3 4	Step R/f backward Hop R/f Step L/f backward Hop L/f Arms slowly come down as both groups return to form the original circle.	Step L/f forward Hop L/f Step R/f forward Hop R/f
	22—24		Repeat of bars 17—20 but with group 'a' taking the part of group 'b', ie coming out of the circle, and 'b' taking the part of 'a', ie going into the circle.	
C	25—28		As 'b's come back from the centre of the circle they turn to their R to meet an 'a' partner. Both link R arms and skip or 'pivot' around in a clockwise direction with the free arm raised high above the head. Keep hips close to each and lean away from each other.	
	29—32		Change arms and go the other way round, ie anti-clockwise. Finish in place ready to move off once again holding the hands of the person either side of you.	

5. *Let There Be Love*

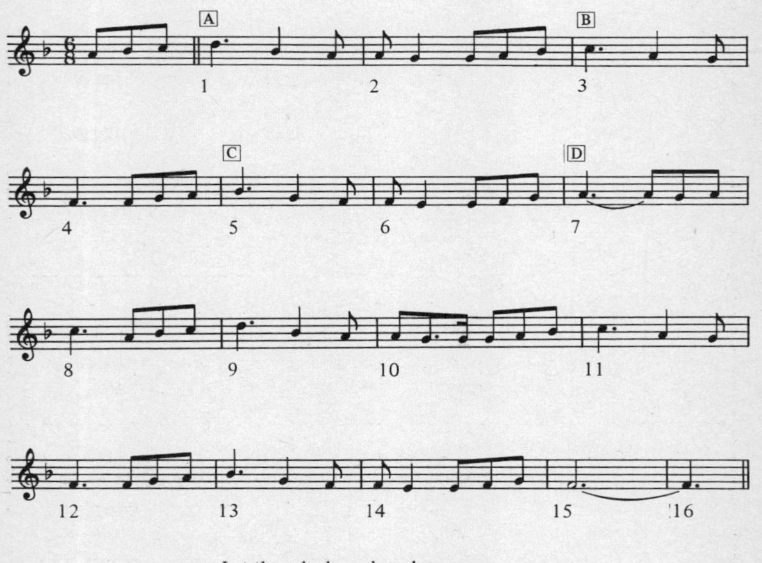

Let there be love shared among us,
Let there be love in our eyes,
May now Your love sweep this nation,
Cause us O Lord to arise.
Give us a fresh understanding
Of brotherly love that is real,
Let there be love shared among us,
Let there be love.

Dave Bilbrough. © 1979 Thankyou Music, P.O. Box 75, Eastbourne BN23 6NW. *SoF 318*

MUSIC	BAR	BEAT	MOVEMENT
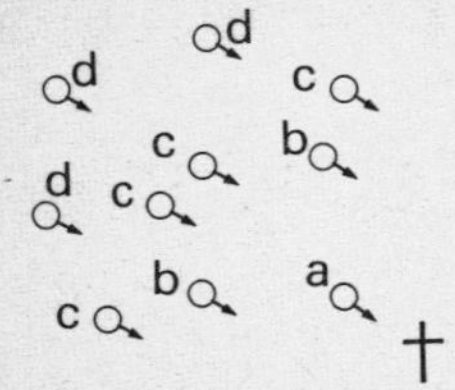			**Starting position** Each dancer, identified as 'a', 'b', 'c' or 'd', stands quietly in the placings suggested. Arms are held loosely at the side of the body. The face is tilted upwards, the eyes focusing on an imaginary cross.
			Motif one 'Let there be love shared among us'
A	1–2		Take the R/l back and slowly sink to kneel on the R/knee. As you do so, bring the arms across the chest with the wrists crossed but not in contact, the palms of the hands facing you. As you come to kneel, lower the head. NB Take a long step back to provide a secure base for the next motif.
			Motif two 'Let there be love in our eyes'
B	3		Stretch the arms out before you, still with wrists crossed and palms upturned. Stretch the torso forward at the same time.
	4		Then open wide to the side, just in front of the body. This should be a warm and generous movement expression combining an attitude of giving oneself and opening oneself wholly. Lean forward with the chest leading high and the head once again focused on the cross.

MUSIC	BAR	BEAT	MOVEMENT
C	5–6		**Motif three** 'May now Your love sweep this nation' Slowly, by taking the weight of the body forward onto the left leg, come to stand tall and slowly bring the arms up high and wide above the head—again slightly forward of the body, with palms upturned, the whole in an attitude of praise.
D	7–8		**Motif four** 'Cause us O Lord to arise' With the arms raised, quietly turn to your right, on the spot, gradually lowering the arms to the side and coming to stand as for the beginning, ready to take the R/l back and sink.
	9–16		Repeat the whole.

The suggested placing is only one of many possibilities, and the dance team should feel free to experiment with other structures. The present plan of facing diagonally forward towards the congregation allows the best possible view of the dance. Normally the cross would be behind the dancer. It may be that you prefer to face the cross or, better still, combine both ideas.

The dance may be performed in unison or four-part canon, either at a one-bar distance or two-bar distance. The dancers, identified as 'a', 'b', 'c' and 'd', enter one after the other in canon at a one-bar or two-bar distance. In effect all four groups will be doing something different at the same time. The effect is very good, both spiritually and aesthetically. Better still, why not combine unison with the two canons?

Whatever you decide, I would suggest that you perform this dance five times: two times sung by all and three times performed by an instrumental combination to produce the following formal structure:

(1) Sung by the congregation and performed by the dancers as instructed, possibly in unison.

(2) Instrumental variation—during this the dancers greet each other in the 'peace' thus reinforcing the narrative by actually doing what it describes.

Towards the end of this first instrumental variation, return to your original 'placings' ready to perform the dance once again, possibly in a developed canonic form.

(3) Sung by congregation with dancers dancing as (1).

(4) Instrumental variation—during this the dancers go into the congregation and encourage the whole church to open up in love towards one another. This instrumental variation may be repeated as many times as necessary for such a happening.

6. *Open Our Eyes, Lord*

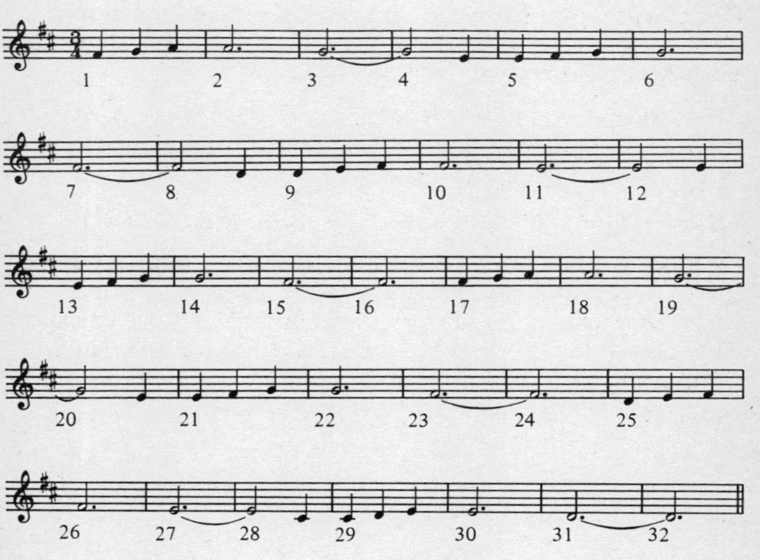

Open our eyes, Lord,
We want to see Jesus,
To reach out and touch Him
And say that we love Him.
Open our ears, Lord,
And help us to listen,
Open our eyes Lord,
We want to see Jesus.

MUSIC	BAR	BEAT	MOVEMENT
	✝		**Starting position** Dancers, carefully placed, kneel back on the R/leg, with arms crossed at the wrists in front of the chest and heads lowered.
	1–8		'Open our eyes, Lord, we want to see Jesus' In unison, the heads come up very slowly to gaze eventually high on the cross.
	9–12		'to reach out and touch Him' In unison, arms are stretched out before one. The wrists remain crossed.
	13–16		'and say that we love Him' In unison the arms open out wide to the side, just slightly in front of the body. Gradually bring the weight of the body onto the L/leg ready to rise.
	17–20		'Open our ears Lord' In unison all slowly rise.
	21–24		'and help us to listen' In unison slowly lift the arms from away to the sides to high and wide above the head.
	25–28		'Open our eyes, Lord' Lower arms.
	29–32		Slowly sink, returning to original position.

I suggest that this dance is performed in the following way:

(1) Sung quietly by all.
(2) Sung and danced.
(3) Quiet instrumental interlude—meditation.
(4) Sung and danced.
(5) Hummed very quietly—end in silence and stillness.

7. *Jesus, How Lovely You Are*

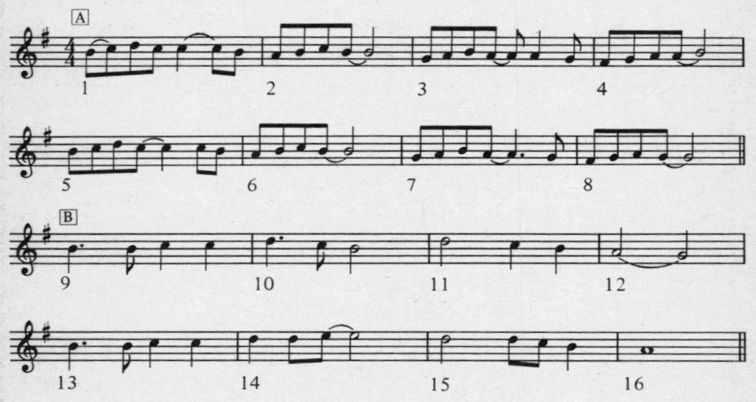

Jesus, how lovely You are,
You are so gentle so pure and kind.
You shine as the morning star,
Jesus, how lovely You are.

1. Hallelujah, Jesus is my Lord and King;
Hallelujah, Jesus is my everything.

2. Hallelujah, Jesus died and rose again;
Hallelujah, Jesus forgave all my sin.

3. Hallelujah, Jesus is meek and lowly;
Hallelujah, Jesus is pure and holy.

4. Hallelujah, Jesus is the Bridegroom;
Hallelujah, Jesus will take His Bride soon.

Dave Bolton. © 1975 Thankyou Music, P.O. Box 75, Eastbourne BN23 6NW. *SoF 274*

MUSIC	BAR	BEAT	MOVEMENT
			Starting position Dancers, identified as 'a' and 'b' alternately, stand in a circle facing centre with hands in contact and held low, ready to move to the left, facing L.
A	1	1 3	**Chorus** Step L/f forward Step R/f forward
	2	1 3 4	Step L/f forward Step R/f back Bend R/knee
	3	1 3	Step L/f forward Step R/f forward
	4	1 3 4	Step L/f forward Step R/f back Bend R/knee
	5	1 3	Step L/f forward Step R/f forward
	6	1 3 4	Step L/f forward Step R/f back Bend R/knee
	7	1 3	Step L/f forward Step R/f forward
	8	1 3 4	Step L/f forward Step R/f back Bend R/knee...

This is a very gentle, unhurried motif. On the second and fourth beats of each bar let the knee give slightly to produce a relaxed bounce. The knee bend on the fourth beat of bars 2, 4, 6 and 8 should be a little more pronounced.

...release hands and turn to face centre of circle.

MUSIC	BAR	BEAT	MOVEMENT	
			'a'	**'b'**
B	9	1 3	Step L/f forward Step R/f forward	Step L/f forward Step R/f forward
	10	1 3	Step L/f forward Step R/f forward Step forward into the centre of circle. As you do so bring the arms across the front of the body—R/arm over L/arm— and up high and wide above the head in a gesture of praise and thanksgiving.	Step L/f forward Step R/f forward Step out of the main circle to produce your own small circle on the spot—moving away to the R. As you do so, let the arms come up high and wide above the head in a gesture of praise and thanksgiving.
	11	1 3	Step L/f back Step R/f back	'Pivot Turn'—on R/f to the R. As you do so slowly, lower the arms until they come down to the side.
	12	1 3	Step L/f back Step R/f back As you retreat slowly lower arms outwards and down to the side.	

MUSIC	BAR	BEAT	MOVEMENT	
	13	1	Step L/f forward	Step L/f forward
		3	Step R/f forward	Step R/f forward
	14	1	Step L/f forward	Step L/f forward
		3	Step R/f forward	Step R/f forward
			Step out of the main circle to produce your own circle on the spot, moving away to the R. As you do so let your arms come up high and wide above your head in a gesture of praise and thanks-giving.	Step forward into the centre of the circle. As you do so bring the arms across the front of the body—R/arm over L and up, high and wide above the head in a gesture of praise and thanks-giving.
	15	1	'Pivot turn'—on	Step L/f back
		3	R/f to R	Step R/f back
	16	1		Step L/f back
		3		Step R/f back
			All slowly lower arms while moving.	
			All be prepared to join hands once again and return to the Chorus.	

The Chorus motif—three steps forward and one step back, may be used for the whole song and performed as a farandole by the whole congregation.

Another interesting idea with regard to this song is to do the whole in double time. At the moment the dance moves on the first and third beats but it could move on all four beats—with an exuberant and lively effect. For example:

MUSIC	BAR	BEAT	MOVEMENT
A	1	1	Step L/f side L
		&	Close R/f to L
		2	Step L/f side L
		&	Close R/f to L
		3	Step L/f side L
		&	Close R/f to L
		4	Step L/f side L
		&	Hop L/f
	2	1	Step R/f side R
		&	Close L/f to R
		2	Step R/f side R
		&	Close L/f to R
		3	Step R/f side R
		&	Close L/f to R
		4	Step R/f side R
		&	Hop R/f
			Release hands.
	3	1	Step L/f forward
		2	Step R/f forward
		3	Step L/f forward
		4	Step R/f forward
			As you step into the circle bring the arms across the body and up high and wide above the head in a movement of praise.
	4	1	Step L/l back
		2	Step R/l back
		3	Step L/l back
		4	Step R/f back
			As you step back out of the circle slowly bring the arms down.
	5–8		Repeat bars 1–4
	13–16		Repeat bars 9–12

8. *Holy Is the Lord*

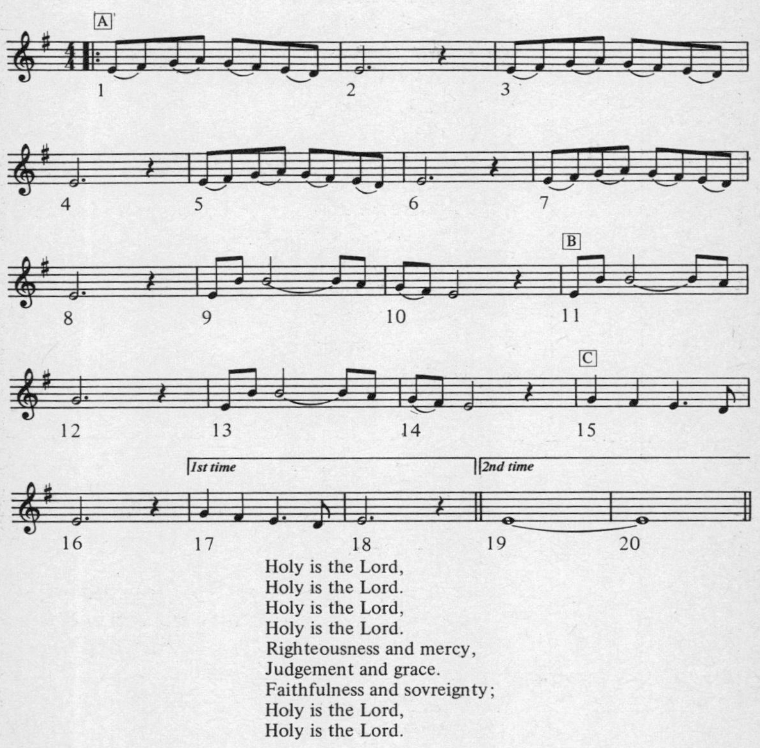

Kelly Green. © 1982 Mercy Publishing.
Administered in Europe by Thankyou Music, P.O. Box 75, Eastbourne BN23 6NW. *SoF 170*

MUSIC	BAR	BEAT	MOVEMENT
			Starting position Dancers identified as 'a' and 'b'—if possible, male and female—stand quiet and still before the cross.
A	1		'a's take their R/l back and slowly sink onto the R knee, at the same time lowering the head, taking up a posture of reverence and awe.
	2		'b's as above.
	3		'a's slowly lift the head and upper torso in adoration and faith.
	4		'b's as above.
	5		'a's tilt the upper torso well forward, letting the arms open away from the side and slightly behind. The head is lowered. The whole is a posture of submission.
	6		'b's as above.
	7		'a's, taking their body weight onto the L/l, slowly come to stand.
	8		'b's as above.

MUSIC	BAR	BEAT	MOVEMENT
B	9	1	'a's raise their arms high and wide above the head by moving from a diagonally forward low position.
		3	'b's raise their arms as above, beginning on the third beat and following two beats behind the 'a's.
	10	1	'a's lower arms, keeping them wide and diagonally slightly forward of the body.
		3	'b's as above.
	11	1	'a's raise their arms high and wide as above
		3	'b's as above.
	12	1	'a's lower arms as in bar 10.
		3	'b's lower arms as in bar 10.
	13	1	'a's raise their arms high and wide as above
		3	'b's as above.
	14	1	'a's lower arms as in bar 10.
		3	'b's lower arms as in bar 10.
	15–16		Stand quietly still.

Go back to the beginning. On the completion of the second time, ie the last two bars of the song, each dancer slowly sinks to his knees. Let this conclusion of the dance continue into the silence.

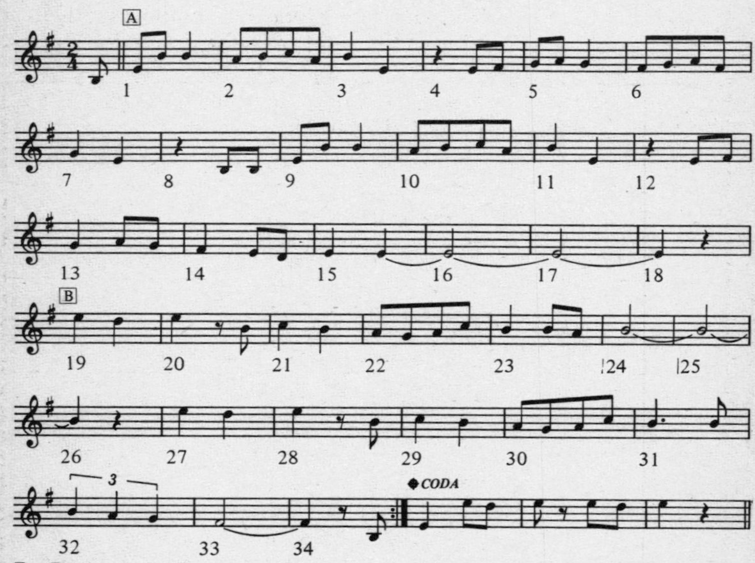

9. *For Zion's Sake*

For Zion's sake I will not keep silent,
For Jerusalem I will not keep quiet,
Till her righteousness goes forth like
  brightness,
Like a flaming torch her salvation.

You will be a crown of beauty
In the hand of the Lord,
You will be a royal diadem
In the hand of your God.

The nations will see your righteousness,
And all kings will see your glory,
And you will be called by a new name
Which the mouth of the Lord will
  choose.

So take no rest for yourselves,
All you who remind the Lord,
And give Him no rest until He makes
Jerusalem a praise in the earth.

MUSIC	BAR	BEAT	MOVEMENT
			Starting position
			The dancers, identified as 'a' and 'b' alternately, form a circle, facing centre, with arms held at shoulder level and hands or palms held loosely in contact ready to move to the left with the grapevine step.
A	1	1 2	Step R/f across L/f Step L/f side L
	2	1 2	Step R/f behind L/f Step L/f side L
	3	1 2	Step R/f across L/f Step L/f side L
	4	1 2	Step R/f behind L/f Step L/f side L
	5	1 2	Step R/f across L/f Step L/f side L
	6	1 2	Step R/f behind L/f Step L/f side L
	7	1 2	Step R/f across L/f Step *back* on L/f behind } mark time
	8	1 2	Step R/f across L/f Hop on R/f
	9	1 2	Step L/f behind R/f Step R/f to R

MUSIC	BAR	BEAT	MOVEMENT
	10	1 2	Step L/f across R/f Step R/f to R
	11	1 2	Step L/f behind R/f Step R/f to R
	12	1 2	Step L/f across R/f Step back behind L/f
	13	1 2	Step L/f small individual half- Step R/f circle walk to the L.
	14	1 2	Step L/f (keep weight on L/f in order to:) Stamp R/f
	15	1 2	Step R/f to R Close L/f to R/f
	16	1 2	Step R/f to R Close L/f to R/f
	17	1 2	Step R/f to R } pivot turn on the R/f to Close L/f to R/f the R. Arms high and
	18	1 2	Step R/f to R Hop R/f
B	19	1 2	Stamp! L/f forward Stamp! R/f forward
	20	1 2	Stamp! L/f forward Hop R/f

Bars 15–18: pivot turn on the R/f to the R. Arms high and wide above the head in an expression of praise. Bring down slowly.

Bars 19–20: Advance into the circle centre, clapping in time with the stamping, bringing the hands high above the head.

MUSIC	BAR	BEAT	MOVEMENT
	21	1	Step L/f back Hop L/f
		2	Step R/f back Hop R/f
	22	1	Step L/f back Hop L/f
		2	Step R/f back Hop R/f

On retreating, let the arms come slowly down from high and wide above the head as you skip back.

'a's turn to their left and 'b's turn to their right and come to face each other. Each hooks the R arm of the other and runs round in a clockwise direction.

MUSIC	BAR	BEAT	MOVEMENT
	23	1	Step R/f forward
		2	Step L/f forward
	24	1	Step R/f forward
		2	Step L/f forward

'arming' to the R

MUSIC	BAR	BEAT	MOVEMENT
	25	1	Step R/f forward
		2	Step L/f forward
	26	1	Step R/f forward
		2	Hop R/f
	27	1	Stamp! L/f forward
		2	Stamp! R/f forward
	28	1	Stamp! L/f forward
		2	Hop L/f

Advance into the circle centre, clapping in time with the stamping bringing the hands high above the head.

On retreating, let the arms come slowly down from high and wide above the head.

MUSIC	BAR	BEAT	MOVEMENT
	29	1	Step L/f back Hop L/f
		2	Step R/f back Hop R/f
	30	1	Step L/f back Hop L/f
		2	Step R/f back Hop R/f
			'a's turn to their left and 'b's turn to their right, facing each other. Each hooks the L arm of the other and runs round in an anticlockwise direction. The free arm is raised high above the head.
	31	1	Step L/f forward
		2	Step R/f forward
	32	1	Step L/f forward — arming to the L
		2	Step R/f forward
	33	1	Step L/f forward
		2	Step R/f forward
	34	1	Step L/f forward
		2	Hop L/f — Release partner and come quickly to face circle centre, ready to go back to the beginning.

MUSIC	BAR	BEAT	MOVEMENT	
Coda	35	1	Step R/f across L	A small individual circle on the spot to the R, ending with a stamp of the R foot. Arms in the air, high and wide.
		2	Step L/f forward	
	36	1	Step R/f forward	
		2	Step L/f forward	
	37	1	Stamp! R/f	

Throughout the whole of this dance, keep the upper torso held high, don't let the head look down at the feet. On the contrary, let the head move to the left 'high' when the R/f comes across, and let the head move to the right 'high' when it comes behind the L/f as you travel L. Similarly when going to the R, let the head move opposite to the working leg.

During the arming motif, pull away from each other but keep in contact hip to hip. Hold the free arm high above the head. Make the 'hops' and 'skips' joyful and bouncy.

As with all the dances shown here, please feel free to develop or simplify. The ideas here are initial suggestions and are meant to encourage you to make up your own dances.

10. *Holy, Holy, Holy Is the Lord*

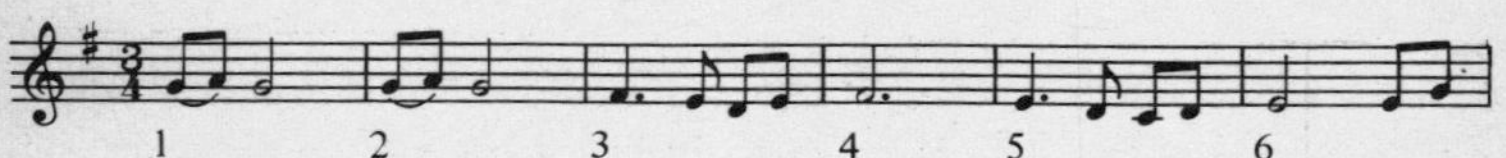

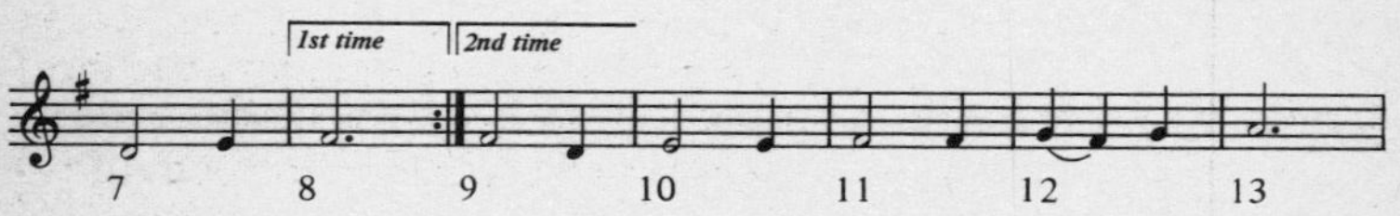

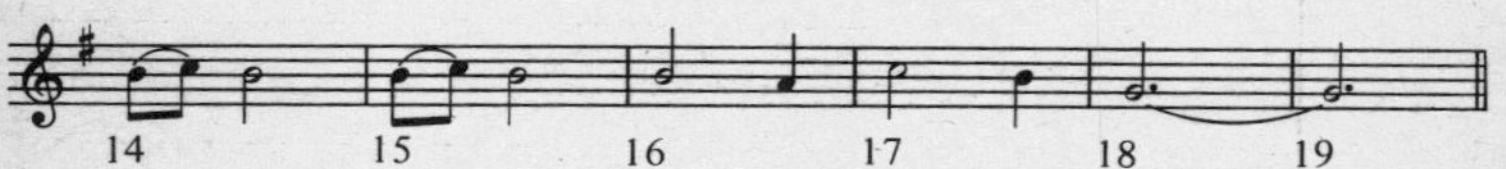

Holy, Holy, Holy is the Lord,
Holy is the Lord God Almighty.
Holy, Holy, Holy is the Lord,
Holy is the Lord God Almighty.
Who was and is and is to come,
Holy, Holy, Holy is the Lord.

Worthy, worthy, worthy is . . . (etc.)

Jesus, Jesus, Jesus is ... . (etc.)

Glory, glory, glory to . . . (etc.)

Author unknown. *SoF 166*

MUSIC	BAR	BEAT	MOVEMENT
			Starting position Dancers, identified as 'a', 'b' and 'c', stand, with feet together, quietly gazing up at the cross. Arms are held loosely at the side.
			Motif A1 'Holy, holy, holy is the Lord! Slowly, at one bar intervals, ie in canon, each group in turn takes the R/l back and slowly comes to kneel on the R knee. At the same time the arms are brought up to the chest with wrists crossed but not in contact and held slightly away from the body. The head is lowered.
A1	1		Group 'a' kneels.
	2		Group 'b' kneels.
	3		Group 'c' kneels.
	4		Hold still.
B1	5–8		'Holy is the Lord God Almighty.' All, in unison, slowly bring the head up to gaze high upon the cross.
			Motif A2 'Holy, holy, holy is the Lord' Slowly, at one-bar intervals, ie in canon, each group in turn stretches out the arms with wrists crossed before them. Keep the face focused high on the cross.

MUSIC	BAR	BEAT	MOVEMENT
A2	1		Group 'a' reaches forward.
	2		Group 'b' reaches forward.
	3		Group 'c' reaches forward.
	4		Hold still.
B2	5–8		**Motif B2** 'Holy is the Lord God Almighty' All, in unison, slowly open the arms wide out to the side, ending up with them slightly diagonally forward of the body, palms upturned.
C	9–12		**Motif C** 'Who was and is and is to come' Slowly, at one bar intervals, each group in turn brings their weight onto the L/l and comes to stand tall, with arms held loosely at the side, and head held high focusing on the cross.
D	13–15		**Motif D** 'Holy, holy, holy is the Lord' In unison, all slowly bring the arms up from the side to wide and high above the head, just slightly forward of the shoulders.
	16–18		In unison, all slowly bring the arms down and return to the original position ready for the repeat from the beginning.

Dance placing

The actual positioning of the dance and dancers is as important as dance steps. Frequently this aspect of choreography is negelected or taken for granted. The careful placing of the dancers both as individuals and as a group is an important consideration, as is the nature of the physical space within which the dance is to be performed.

Some possibilities for 'placing' are illustrated below. You might find some of these 'placings' more appropriate than the ones suggested for each enclosed dance.

1

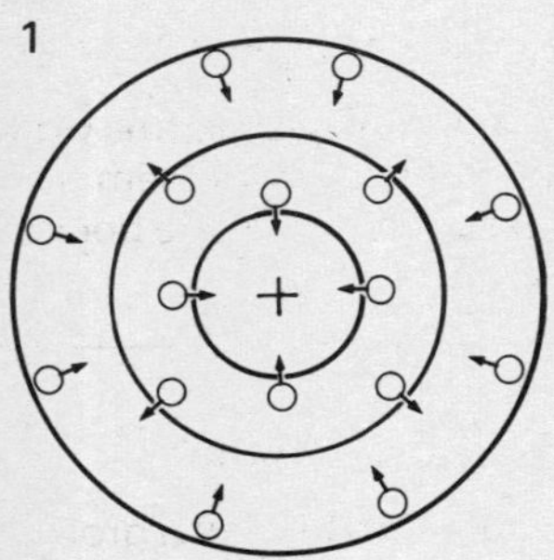

2

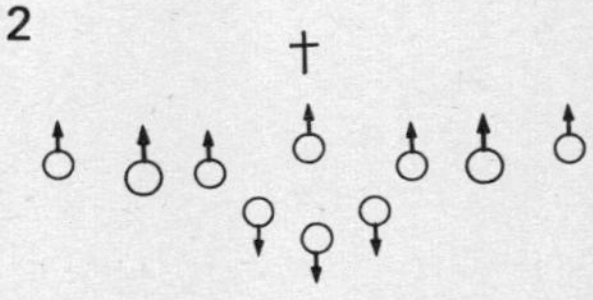

Consider the possibility of dancers facing in different directions, eg (1) and (3).

3

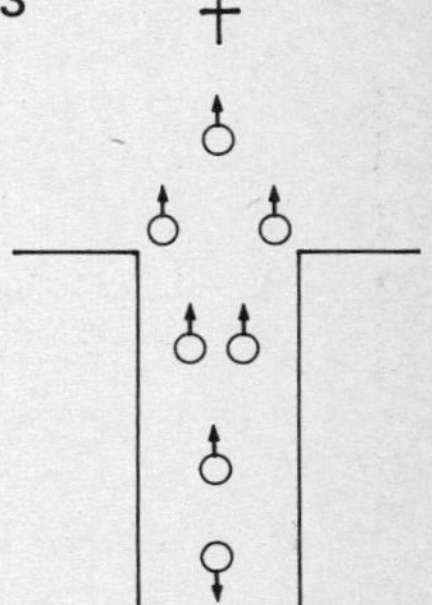

4

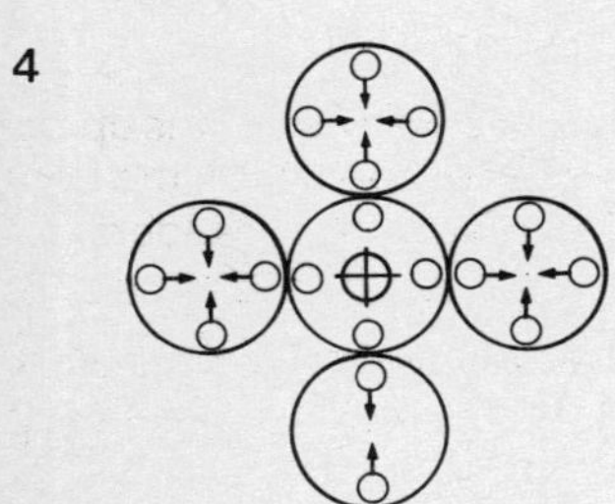

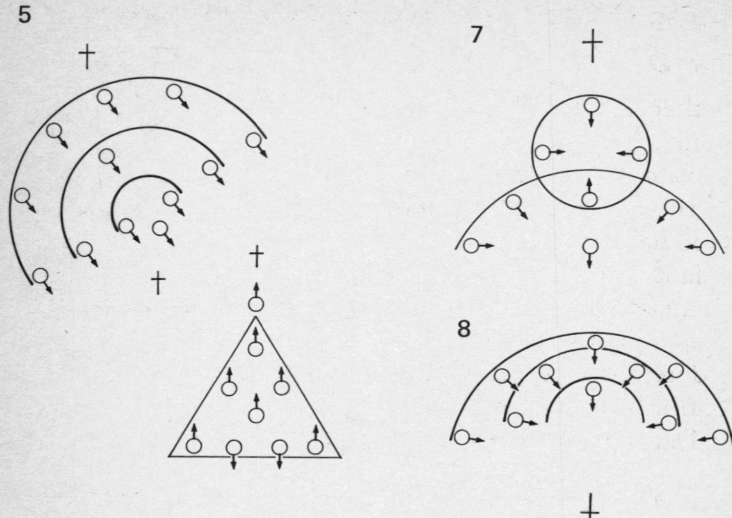

Consider the use of different levels, eg (4)—the centre group could be on a raised level, or (1)—all three circles could be on a different level, or (3) the leader could be on a higher level.

Many of the dances shown here can be performed to other well-known spiritual songs. The reader is encouraged to experiment with adapting some of the dances. The following represent some fairly simple adaptations:

(1) 'We really want to thank you Lord' goes well with 'I will enter His gates'.

(2) 'Let there be love' goes well with 'Jesus, Name above all names' and 'Sing Hallelujah to the Lord'.

(3) 'Open our eyes, Lord' goes well with 'River wash over me'.

(4) 'Jubilate Deo' goes well with 'Bring a psalm'.

Other spiritual songs choreographed by the author:

Time to Dance (Collins: London, 1984).

> Father we adore You
> Sing to our Father
> Salvator mundi (music from Taizé)
> In the presence of Your people
> God has spoken
> Infant holy
> Ding dong merrily on high ⎫ three Christmas carols
> Quem pastores laudavere ⎭
> Adoremus Te Domine II (music from Taizé)
> Gloria (music from Taizé)
> A Dance Project (based on Psalm 95)

Dance and the Christian Faith (Hodder and Stoughton: London, 1985).

> Angelus ad Virginem (Christmas carol)
> Broken for me
> Jesus came to die on a tree
> There's a quiet understanding
> Turn your eyes upon Jesus
> Holy, holy, holy Lord
> The Lord is present
> God has spoken
> Ostende nobis (music from Taizé)
> Creative Dance Projects
> 'Gloria' (Vivaldi)
> The Prayer of Humble Access ('La Nottee': Vivaldi)
> The wondrous cross (music — Ave Verum: Byrd)

An audio cassette specifically designed to accompany the above dances is available from Collins in the case of *Time to Dance*, and 'Christian Sound Services', 43 Linden Road, Enfield, Middlesex, in the case of *Dance and The Christian Faith*.